Core Assessment and Training

Human Kinetics

with

Jason Brumitt
MSPT, SCS, ATC, CSCS*D

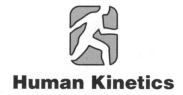

Human Kinetics

Library of Congress Cataloging-in-Publication Data

Core assessment and training / Human Kinetics with Jason Brumitt.
    p. ; cm.
  Includes bibliographical references and index.
  ISBN-13: 978-0-7360-7384-4 (soft cover)
  ISBN-10: 0-7360-7384-1 (soft cover)
  1. Physical education and training. 2. Abdomen----Muscles. 3. Chest--Muscles. I. Brumitt, Jason. II. Human Kinetics (Organization)
  [DNLM: 1. Exercise. 2. Physical Fitness. 3. Athletic Injuries--prevention & control. 4. Athletic Injuries--rehabilitation. 5. Exercise Therapy--methods. 6. Musculoskeletal System--injuries. QT 255 C797 2010]
  GV711.5.C662 2010
  613.7--dc22

                      2009036254

ISBN-10: 0-7360-7384-1
ISBN-13: 978-0-7360-7384-4

The Web addresses cited in this text were current as of October, 2009, unless otherwise noted.

Acquisitions Editor: Melinda Flegel; **Developmental Editor:** Kathleen Bernard; **Managing Editor:** Katherine Maurer; **Assistant Editors:** Nicole Gleeson, Steven Calderwood, and Elizabeth Evans; **Copyeditor:** Patrick Connolly; **Indexer:** Nancy Ball; **Permission Manager:** Dalene Reeder; **Graphic Designer:** Joe Buck; **Graphic Artist:** Denise Lowry; **Cover Designer:** Keith Blomberg; **Photographer (cover and interior):** Neil Bernstein; **Photo Asset Manager:** Laura Fitch; **Visual Production Assistant:** Joyce Brumfield; **Photo Production Manager:** Jason Allen; **Art Manager:** Kelly Hendren; **Associate Art Manager:** Alan L. Wilborn; **Illustrator:** Jason M. McAlexander, MFA; **Printer:** Versa Press

Printed in the United States of America   10 9 8 7 6 5 4 3 2

The paper in this book is certified under a sustainable forestry program.

Human Kinetics
Web site: www.HumanKinetics.com

United States: Human Kinetics, P.O. Box 5076, Champaign, IL 61825-5076
800-747-4457
e-mail: humank@hkusa.com

Canada: Human Kinetics, 475 Devonshire Road Unit 100, Windsor, ON N8Y 2L5
800-465-7301 (in Canada only)
e-mail: info@hkcanada.com

Europe: Human Kinetics, 107 Bradford Road, Stanningley, Leeds LS28 6AT, United Kingdom
+44 (0) 113 255 5665
e-mail: hk@hkeurope.com

Australia: Human Kinetics, 57A Price Avenue, Lower Mitcham, South Australia 5062
08 8372 0999
e-mail: info@hkaustralia.com

New Zealand: Human Kinetics, P.O. Box 80, Torrens Park, South Australia 5062
0800 222 062
e-mail: info@hknewzealand.com

E4406

Contents

Preface

Core training is one of the hottest trends in fitness and rehabilitation. Our understanding of the role that the core plays in health, injury prevention, sport performance, and rehabilitation has grown dramatically in recent years. Furthermore, biomechanists and sports medicine researchers are continually advancing this understanding—new breakthroughs are occurring all the time. What was true 10 years ago is not true today!

Unfortunately, the terms *core assessment* and *core training* are sometimes thrown around as a catchall phrase describing any exercise or series of exercises purported to train this region of the body. The concepts of core stability training are often misunderstood, resulting in training programs that are poorly designed and sometimes dangerous.

Whether you are a personal trainer, a strength coach, or a rehabilitation professional, you must be able to properly analyze core function and be able to implement safe and effective training programs. This will enable you to help your clients maximize their goals.

To aid your understanding of key core assessments and exercises, the accompanying DVD includes video demonstrations that review proper techniques for many of the exercises and assessments. Throughout the text, assessments and exercises that are demonstrated on the DVD are marked with a DVD icon. A complete list of the assessments and exercises on the DVD appears on page 154.

No two people are the same, and the training programs for two people should not be the same either! *Core Assessment and Training* will help you improve your ability to assess a client's baseline core function. This book will also help you develop the best individualized program for each of your clients.

1

Introduction to Core Training

itness and sports medicine professionals share the common goal of developing and implementing optimal training programs for their clients and athletes. Billions of dollars are spent each year by individuals, schools, universities, and professional teams in order to build better athletes and improve sport and human performance. Likewise, thousands of people employ the services of personal trainers each year in an effort to improve their health and physical fitness. Despite the pursuit of optimal sport performance or improved physical fitness, people who exercise (let alone those who do not exercise) are not immune to injury.

THE CHALLENGE OF DESIGNING OPTIMAL TRAINING PROGRAMS

With all of the technological advances and training innovations designed to enhance sport and human performance, one might assume that the risk of a sport- or work-related overuse injury would be a thing of the past. Unfortunately, this is not the case. Physicians' offices, emergency rooms, physical therapy clinics, and athletic training centers are often filled with competitive athletes, weekend warriors, and laborers seeking care for musculoskeletal injuries. Billions of dollars in health care costs are incurred each year by Americans requiring medical treatment for musculoskeletal injuries.

Injuries to the low back (or low back pain) account for the majority of musculoskeletal injuries. The economic costs associated with low back pain are staggering. In the United States over $25 billion is spent each year treating patients who are suffering from low back pain (Luo et al. 2004).

The total economic cost (health care costs, loss of work time, loss of productivity) related to low back pain has been estimated to be nearly $200 billion annually in the United States (Katz 2006).

Millions of patients receive conservative treatments from practitioners such as physical therapists, athletic trainers, chiropractors, and massage therapists. Patients who fail to improve with conservative measures may require more extensive medical evaluations (including imaging studies), the prescription of pain or anti-inflammatory medications, and invasive treatments such as injections or surgery. These medical treatments are not without risk. Radiographs (X rays) expose the body to radiation, prescription medications may cause negative side effects, and surgical interventions sometimes fail to alleviate the person's pain. Despite the resources devoted to the diagnosis and treatment of low back pain, optimal treatment strategies continue to elude health care providers. The best treatment strategy may be to prescribe a comprehensive exercise program that focuses on training the core.

Why Athletes and Fitness Clients Still Sustain Injuries

Why are athletes still sustaining injuries? A likely reason is the inadequate design of the athlete's strength training program, including a failure to address all potential risk factors for injury. When developing and implementing strength training programs, many training professionals rely on their own past experiences or on the advice of an exercise "guru." Using past experiences or suggestions from training experts (who often rely on their own past experiences) may be helpful in guiding the initial development of a program.

However, these routines may fail to account for one or more key components of a comprehensive training program. For training professionals who are seeking assistance with program design, a better option is to access the research literature. Unfortunately, many times there is a **paucity** (or a lack) of good research to help guide the decisions on program design. This book highlights evidence-based training programs (when available). In addition, evidence-supported strategies are presented to help coaches, fitness professionals, and sports medicine practitioners design and implement optimal core training programs. These strategies enable program designers to fill in the gaps in the research literature so they can create effective programs for their clients.

Should a female cross country athlete perform the same strength training program as a male football player? Obviously not. However, some athletes are prescribed a "one-size-fits-all" training program. Although some similar exercises may be performed by different athletic populations, the design of the athlete's training program should be guided by the physiological requirements of the sport as well as the strength and conditioning needs of the individual. In addition, an appreciation for injury risk factors and the proper mechanics of the sport should be factored into the final exercise program.

To highlight the challenges of using the research literature when developing a strength training program, let's look at the female high school athlete in the sport of cross country. Endurance runners risk injury to any lower extremity joint. **Epidemiological** investigations of high school cross country runners have found that female cross country athletes have a greater risk of sustaining a sport-related lower extremity injury when compared with their male counterparts (Rauh et al. 2000; Rauh et al. 2006). Once injured, a majority of the athletes were able to return to running after being sidelined for 1 to 4 days. Although this time lost to injury may seem short, it becomes significant if the injury occurs a day or two before a meet. Also of significance is the finding that, once injured, the cross country athlete has a four- to fivefold increase in her chances of reinjuring the same body part during the season.

Once it has been demonstrated that a particular population—in this case, the female cross country athlete—is at risk (or has a greater risk of injury than another group), potential risk factors should be investigated. Numerous risk factors have been proposed as having a role in the onset of a running-related injury, but very few published reports exist that support (or refute) these claims. An epidemiological investigation was conducted to determine the incidence of **medial tibial stress syndrome (MTSS)** in cross country athletes at the high school level and to identify potential risk factors associated with this injury (Plisky et al. 2007). Some of the risk factors analyzed in this investigation included sex, **body mass index (BMI),** running experience, navicular drop (an objective measurement of foot mechanics), and history of running injury. Female cross country athletes experienced a greater incidence of MTSS and only one risk factor (a higher BMI) demonstrated an association with an increased risk of a MTSS injury.

Findings from this type of epidemiological report should influence strength training coaches who design training programs for cross country athletes at the high school level. However, this athletic population—female high school athletes in the sport of cross country—provides an example of a paucity in the literature regarding each potential factor that may increase the risk of injury (these factors may include hip weakness, poor core endurance capacity, and asymmetrical range of motion in the hip and lumbar area). Because of the lack of epidemiological investigations that assess all potential risk factors, designing and implementing training programs that reduce the risk of injury can be a challenge.

When there is a lack of research (in this case, a lack of epidemiological reports and **evidence-based** training programs), professionals should look for additional studies and reports that use similar populations (e.g., college runners instead of high school runners). These complementary reports may improve one's ability to design a program for the female cross country athlete at the high school level.

In one such study, a **handheld dynamometer** was used to objectively measure the strength of six hip muscle groups in 30 recreational runners (ranging in age from 18 to 55) who were diagnosed with a unilateral running-related overuse injury (Niemuth et al. 2005). The researchers compared these findings with a control group of uninjured runners. They found no significant differences in hip strength between the control group and the uninvolved hip of the injured runners. However, within the experimental group (the injured runners), significant weakness was found for the hip abductors and flexors on the injured side. In addition, the hip adductors were significantly stronger on the injured side. Although a direct cause-and-effect relationship cannot be concluded from this study, the results indicate that hip weakness or muscular imbalance may be associated with running injuries.

In another study, researchers retrospectively identified hip abductor weakness in distance runners with **iliotibial band syndrome (ITBS)** (Fredericson et al. 2000). Runners who had been diagnosed with ITBS demonstrated significant weakness of the hip abductors when compared with uninjured controls. The experimental group was composed of 24 consecutive collegiate or club long-distance runners who attended a "runners' injury clinic" for evaluation and were diagnosed with ITBS. They were compared to a control group consisting of 30 distance runners from Stanford University's cross country or track teams. Those who were diagnosed with ITBS subsequently participated in a 6-week rehab program. The therapy program involved one or two sessions of therapeutic **modalities** along with a progression through a standardized exercise program (consisting of two strengthening exercises for the gluteus medius and two stretching exercises). The injured athletes who participated in the rehab program realized an increase of 35% (females) to 51% (males) in hip abductor torque. Also, 22 of the 24 runners returned to their sport at 6 weeks. This case series is an important study adding to the clinical belief that hip weakness in distance runners may adversely affect biomechanics, thus contributing to overuse-related injuries in the lower extremity.

The findings from these reports suggest that weakness of the core muscles may be a factor in the onset of a running-related injury. Although additional prospective investigations are warranted, the research indicates that a strength training program for this population should address weakness of the core.

Even less research is available to guide exercise prescription for the nonathletic client. A majority of the sports medicine research has focused on the competitive athlete (high school to professional ranks). The literature definitely lacks research related to the recreational athlete or the weekend warrior. In addition, it is difficult to find epidemiological research or evidence-supported training programs for those who work in jobs that involve intensive manual labor. Despite advancements in the field of **ergonomics,** the implementation of corporate injury prevention programs, and employee education on proper lifting mechanics and body awareness, work-related musculoskeletal injuries continue to occur. These injuries contribute to lost productivity, soaring health care costs, and disruption to the lifestyle of the employee.

What Is Missing From Current Programs?

Sometimes athletes and clients fail to follow the training or rehabilitation programs that were designed for them. In some cases, this problem (albeit not a simple one) can be remedied by properly motivating the client (Brown 2004; Middleton 2004; Milne et al. 2005; Muse 2005; Sabin 2005). However, the problem is often the result of the strength training professional (e.g., fitness trainer, strength coach, or sports medicine professional) failing to design and implement a comprehensive training program.

Program design can be extremely challenging. A training professional can feel overwhelmed just trying to figure out where to begin. It would be easy if a universal training program could be prescribed to an individual based on the person's sport or functional goals. The advantage of a "cookbook" program or protocol is that it can offer training suggestions purported to be beneficial by other trainers, coaches, or rehabilitation professionals. Unfortunately, cookbook programs do not account for individual differences in athletes or clients.

The following are clinical cases that represent examples of clients or athletes seen every day in athletic training rooms, rehabilitation clinics, and fitness centers. As you read each scenario, attempt to identify potential functional weaknesses or limitations for each client. Then generate some training ideas to help correct those dysfunctions.

■ **Clinical scenario 1:** A 35-year-old female wants to resume a running program. In the past, she ran to maintain physical fitness. She has also participated in weekend 5K and 10K fun runs in the past and wishes to be able to do that again. She had a cesarean section 4 months ago and has not run in over a year and a half. This client will present with abdominal weakness related to the cesarean and more than likely will also present with muscular weakness or imbalance in the remaining core muscles. Failure to address muscular dysfunction and weakness may contribute to the onset of a lower back or lower extremity running-related injury. The addition of a core training program may help to reduce the risk of sustaining an injury.

■ **Clinical scenario 2:** A high school discus thrower is frequently straining muscles in his low back. He usually experiences an episode of low back pain when he practices longer than 2 hours in a day. He is currently performing a training program (which his coach adopted from a track and field Web site) that includes squats and lunges. He is able to demonstrate adequate power and strength based on the amount of weight he is able to lift, but something is obviously missing. Evaluating the endurance capacity of his core muscles is crucial. Fatigue of these muscles will affect how forces are generated and transferred through his kinetic chain as he throws.

■ **Clinical scenario 3:** A 23-year-old female has suffered pain in the front of both knees for 3 years. Her previous three attempts at physical therapy have failed to reduce her pain or improve her functional ability. She is employed as a medical transcriptionist and is generally sedentary. She continues to do the exercises previously prescribed by her physical therapist: straight leg raises and short arc quads to strengthen the hip flexors and quadriceps, and hamstring stretches. Is a rehab or postrehab program complete if it emphasizes only the quadriceps and hamstrings? There is research suggesting that the hip musculature plays a crucial role in lower extremity biomechanics. Weakness in the hip may dramatically affect the stresses experienced at the knee.

TRAINING THE CORE IS THE MISSING LINK

In the scenarios described in the previous section, the exercise programs likely failed because they were missing one essential component: core training.

Core training, a popular buzzword in the fitness and rehabilitation worlds, is still poorly understood. In the training programs prescribed by some trainers or therapists, the choice of exercises for training the core (or the lack of core exercises) is often shocking. Core stability training should serve as a foundation for all training and rehabilitation programs. Core training *should not* promote or cause dysfunction in clients! Fitness professionals who follow the advice of a training guru may invite trouble for their clients. These trainers may apply the flavor-of-the-month exercise or implement a generic training program for *all* of their clients irrespective of individual needs and goals.

The strategies outlined in this book will help you design and implement evidence-supported core training programs that reduce the risk of injury and maximize the client's performance (sport or functional performance). To develop optimal training programs, you must be able to assess your clients' functional needs, identify their weaknesses, and prescribe the appropriate exercises. This text guides you through the process of assessment, testing, and prescription of core exercises.

DEFINING CORE TRAINING

Before developing a core training program, you must have an understanding of the core and its unique functional roles. The *core* is the region of the body consisting of the muscles and joints of the abdomen, the low back, the pelvis, and the hips. An overview of human skeletal musculature is shown in figure 1.1. (A basic review of functional anatomy is provided in chapter 2.) The core muscles have dual roles. The first role is protecting (stabilizing) the spine from excessive (and potentially injurious) forces; the second role is in the creation and transfer of forces in a proximal-to-distal sequence (Kibler et al. 2006). **Proximal-to-distal sequencing** refers to how a force may be generated or created and then transferred through the body. An easy way to understand proximal-to-distal sequencing is to think of the pitching motion in baseball. As the pitcher begins his windup, he is generating a force with his rear leg. During the pitching motion, this force is transferred from the lower extremity (proximally) through the body to the throwing arm (distally) in order to maximize the velocity of the pitch.

When the core muscles are functioning optimally, the person will be able to safely perform athletic or functional activities. When dysfunction is present, the person's performance will suffer, and she may also be at an increased risk for injury.

Two terms associated with core training are *core stability* and *core stabilization.* These terms relate to the ability of the core muscles to protect the spine (the terms are also used to describe the exercises that promote core stability). Stability of the core (for athletes) has been defined as "the ability to control the position and motion of the trunk over the pelvis to allow optimum production, transfer and control of force and motion to the terminal segment in integrated athletic (or kinetic chain) activities" (Kibler et al. 2006, p. 189). Failure to adequately train these muscles will limit the effectiveness of the core in doing its job. *Core training,* then, is the process of using specific exercises to maximize the core's unique functional roles.

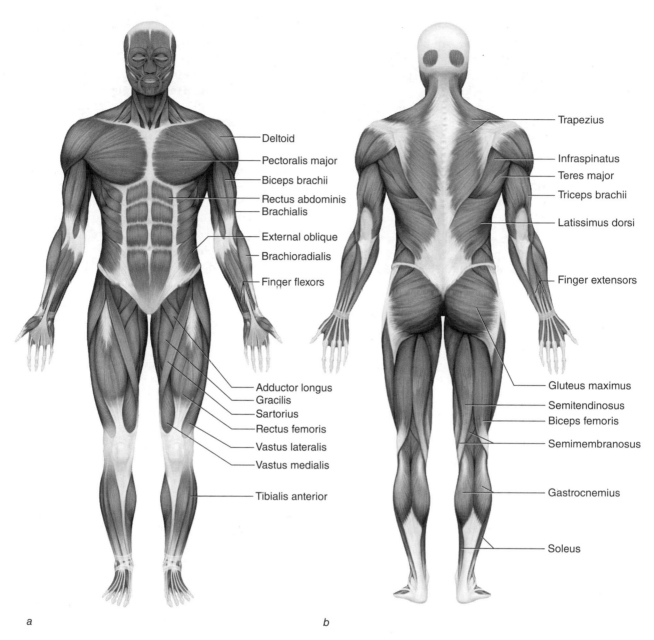

Figure 1.1 Adult male human skeletal musculature, *(a)* front and *(b)* rear views. The core consists of the muscles and joints of the abdomen, low back, pelvis, and hips.

Reprinted, by permission, from NSCA, 2008, Biomechanics of resistance exercise, by E. Harman. In *Essentials of strength training and conditioning,* 3rd ed., edited by T. Baechle and R. Earle (Champaign, IL: Human Kinetics), 68.

How many of your clients are performing basic core exercises? The answer should be all of them. All fitness clients, athletes, rehab patients, and postrehab clients will benefit from the inclusion of core exercises in their individualized training programs.

Improving Physical Fitness

Many clients who seek out services from fitness professionals have only a basic understanding of

core training. For many, their previous core training may have been limited by ignorance. Some may believe that core exercises can only be performed by using that "one-of-a-kind" piece of equipment they saw on a late-night infomercial. For others, training the core is equated with performing machine-based exercises such as the seated row and the lat pull-down. Unfortunately, some people purchase expensive gym memberships for the sole purpose of having access to the machines that are purported to isolate key core muscles. In reality, a majority of clients can perform core exercises without the use of any form of machinery!

The services you provide as a personal trainer or strength coach may be the only health- and fitness-related services sought by some of your clients. If this is the case, you must carefully listen to the unique history and goals of the client. You must consider any conditions that may warrant a referral to a physician or appropriate health care provider. You should then choose sensible exercises that maximize the client's potential.

Warning

In an effort to prevent their clients from becoming bored, some fitness professionals prescribe exercises that either serve no functional purpose or are potentially unsafe. Avoid having your clients perform circus tricks! An example of a circus trick would be having a 55-year-old nonathletic individual performing a pull-down cable exercise while balancing on a single leg on a BOSU. As you will see later in this book, many of the best exercises for promoting core stability are performed either in static postures or in one plane of motion. These exercises require minimal or no special equipment. Making subtle changes to these basic functional exercises will increase the challenge for the client without sacrificing personal safety.

Preventing Injuries and Rehabilitating Clients

As previously mentioned, back injuries are one of the most common conditions treated by medical doctors, osteopaths, physical therapists, and chiropractors. Unfortunately, there is a lack of consensus among medical professionals regarding how to best treat patients who are suffering from back pain. To prevent the onset of a back injury, an ounce of prevention may truly be worth a pound of cure.

Low back pain will affect up to 80% of the U.S. population (Rasmussen-Barr et al. 2003). Some sustain low back injuries as a result of a traumatic event such as a motor vehicle accident or a fall from a height. In these situations, it is unlikely that a strength training routine or injury prevention program could have helped the person avoid injury. On the other hand, a majority of patients who suffer from low back pain develop an injury from repetitively overstressing the joints and muscles of the spine. Many of these injuries may be avoided if an evidence-supported strength training program is in place.

Training professionals need to change the way they view people who perform physically demanding jobs. Just like an athlete, laborers require their bodies to perform at high levels for prolonged periods of time. Based on that alone, people who perform labor-intensive jobs should be considered *industrial* or *occupational athletes.* Athletes are expected to perform exercises to avoid injury and enhance performance. Industrial athletes should do the same. Some employees may receive specialized training programs at progressive organizations and corporations, but this is far from the norm. Developing wellness programs (including core training exercises) for people in physically demanding occupations is an emerging market for strength training professionals.

The rehabilitation program for an injured industrial athlete should include core training, regardless of whether the person has a back injury or an extremity injury. Researchers tested isometric hip strength bilaterally in individuals who had undergone a unilateral knee surgery (Jaramillo et al. 1994). Significant weakness was found in the hip flexors, extensors, abductors, and adductors on the surgical extremity. This report was unable to demonstrate a direct cause-and-effect relationship between hip weakness and the need for a knee surgery; however, the results from this study highlight the importance of addressing the core musculature as part of a comprehensive rehabilitation program.

Significant consequences can be associated with some athletic injuries. Sport-related injuries to the spine or hips may result in a loss of practice or training time, missed competitions, countless hours of rehabilitation, or possibly the end of the athlete's career. A growing body of research highlights how core weakness in athletes can contribute to the onset of a sport-related injury.

In one study, researchers performed a prospective investigation in order to assess the effects of core weakness on the incidence of athletic injury (Leetun et al. 2004). The researchers analyzed preseason measures of hip strength and trunk endurance to determine if a particular score was associated with the onset of a sport-related injury during the season. One hundred forty college athletes from six schools were tested within 2 weeks of beginning practice. Using a dynamometer, the researchers collected isometric values for hip abduction and external rotation. Trunk

Case Example: Injured Worker With Poor Core Endurance and Dysfunctional Movement Patterns

A 42-year-old male with a physically demanding job was referred to physical therapy with a diagnosis of low back pain. His job entailed lifting loads ranging from 25 to 100 pounds (11.3 to 45.4 kg) consistently throughout the day. While attempting a "light lift" (his words) of 50 pounds (22.7 kg), he felt a pop in his back, and he fell to his knees. He described it as "initially an intense pain with muscle spasms throughout his back." He scheduled an appointment with his medical doctor, who prescribed pain medication, rest, and physical therapy.

The patient's first physical therapy appointment was 2 weeks after the onset of the injury. He reported that his symptoms had improved and his pain had significantly decreased. During the interview portion of the physical therapy evaluation, he told the therapist the following: "I'm not sure why I'm here. I'm as strong as an ox; I can lift whatever I want." This patient was equating a good (healthy) back with the ability to lift required work loads. The physical therapist evaluated the patient's strength, finding him to be not only grossly weak through his trunk musculature (poor endurance capacity of the torso muscles) but also functionally weak. He was unable to demonstrate proper squatting and lunging techniques. Because this patient was unable to use his core muscles to stabilize and protect his spine, he was instead using dysfunctional movement patterns whenever he attempted to lift an object. He likely used poor body mechanics each time he performed a lift. Improper lifting techniques, especially with heavy objects, will impart **supraphysiologic** loads to his spine. Over time, tissues will fail, leading to injury and dysfunction.

---

endurance scores were collected using the endurance tests as described by McGill (see chapter 4) (McGill 2002).

The researchers found that female athletes were significantly weaker in the hip abductors, the hip external rotators, and the lateral core endurance measures (lateral endurance test) than their male counterparts (Leetun et al. 2004). Male athletes also tended to be stronger than the female athletes on the remaining tests. Those who experienced an injury during the season demonstrated significant weakness in both hip abduction and hip external rotation. Preseason weakness of the hip external rotators was determined to be the best predictor for athletes who later sustained a lower extremity injury.

In another study, researchers prospectively tested the hip strength (gluteus maximus and medius) in collegiate athletes to determine if hip strength imbalances increased the likelihood of an athlete requiring treatment for low back pain (LBP) (Nadler et al. 2001). Eight percent of all athletes tested (13 of 163) required LBP treatment during the subsequent year. Not surprisingly, 6 of the 13 athletes had a history of LBP. The percentage difference between a female athlete's left and right hip extensor strength was statistically significant as a predictor for the athlete requiring LBP treatment. All other relationships were determined to be insignificant. The researchers concluded that the findings from this study support the notion of a relationship between hip muscle imbalance and the onset of low back pain in female athletes.

Another group of researchers recorded mean and maximal values for the strength of the hip abductor and extensor muscles in 210 (70 female and 140 male) NCAA collegiate athletes (Nadler et al. 2000). These values were recorded during the athletes' preparticipation screening physical. This investigation was performed to determine if a relationship exists between athletes who demonstrate asymmetrical hip strength and those who have a history of low back or lower extremity injury. Female athletes who reported either a lower extremity injury or low back pain the previous year demonstrated a statistically significant side-to-side difference in maximal hip extension strength. Male athletes who reported a history of low back pain or lower extremity injury did not demonstrate side-to-side differences in hip strength.

In a different study, golfers who had a history of low back pain were found to demonstrate significantly less internal and external rotation of the lead hip when compared to golfers with no history of low back pain (Vad et al. 2004). The golfers with a history of low back pain also demonstrated less flexibility in lumbar extension.

The previous examples show that a dysfunctional core may contribute to an athlete experiencing a sport-related back injury. Core stability training may help to reduce the athlete's risk of injury, aid in rehabilitation after an injury, and enhance athletic performance (Chiu 2007).

Enhancing Athletic Performance

Spine stabilization exercises also serve to enhance athletic performance. The trunk is one component of the functional kinetic link system. For example, athletes who perform overhead throwing will generate power from their lower extremities and transfer those forces through the trunk to the upper extremity. This proximal-to-distal sequencing gives the upper extremity the ability to achieve maximal acceleration at the highest possible speed (Kibler 1998). Dysfunctional activation of the trunk musculature may result in poorer athletic performance. A dysfunctional trunk also places the athlete at risk of injuring a distal segment. The baseball pitcher who has a dysfunctional trunk will still attempt to perform at his optimal level late into a game. The forces generated by the legs will be incompletely transferred to the upper extremity. The pitcher will automatically compensate for this by attempting to generate more torque at the shoulder. Repeating this sequence enough times can lead to excessive loads on the shoulder, resulting in a rotator cuff injury. Establishing adequate endurance capacity and strength of the trunk will not only reduce injury risk but will also improve athletic performance.

SUMMARY

By now you should understand the need for including exercises for the core in the training programs for all clients and athletes. Inadequate program design or a failure to include core exercises may limit the effectiveness of an individual's training program. Failure to address core weakness may put a client or athlete at a greater risk of sustaining a sport- or work-related injury. The growing body of research evidence is pointing to the critical role of core training for injury prevention, rehabilitation, and sport and human performance. Throughout this book, evidence-based training and rehabilitation programs are presented (when available). In addition, evidence-supported strategies are presented to help coaches, fitness professionals, and sports medicine practitioners design and implement optimal core training programs. Research related to core training is in its infancy, and no doubt over time publications from sports medicine researchers will improve our ability to design effective and safe core training programs.

This book is divided into four parts. Part I provides the scientific rationale behind core training; part II covers how to assess a client's core strength and flexibility and how to interpret the findings; part III describes how to develop an evidence-supported core training program based on the client's functional weaknesses; part IV provides a review of common core-related musculoskeletal injuries. Each part builds on the others in order to enhance your ability to design optimal programs for core stability training.

2

Functional Anatomy of the Core

The *core* is the central region of the human body, consisting of musculoskeletal structures from the abdomen, the spine, the pelvis, and the hips (Kibler et al 2006). The core functions to generate movement, create and transfer forces, and provide stability. A dysfunctional core may limit a client's or athlete's performance and may increase the risk of sustaining an injury. Fitness professionals must be able to functionally test the client in order to identify a dysfunctional core. A working knowledge of the functional anatomy of the core will enhance your ability to identify weak or tight muscles and improve your ability to recognize dysfunctional movement patterns. Having this knowledge will improve how you design a core training program and enhance your ability to communicate with other professionals.

This chapter provides a review of the basic functional anatomy of the core, highlighting the functional roles of key core muscles in providing stability and movement. This chapter does *not* provide a comprehensive anatomical or biomechanical study of the core. Refer to a college anatomy text for a more comprehensive review. Two additional reference texts (related to the core and anatomy) that all strength training professionals should own are Stuart McGill's *Low Back Disorders: Evidence-Based Prevention and Rehabilitation, Second Edition* (Human Kinetics 2007) and Robert Behnke's *Kinetic Anatomy, Second Edition* (Human Kinetics 2006).

CORE ANATOMY

Good strength coaches and fitness professionals know how to prescribe a strength training or rehabilitation program and how to progress an individual through that program. Great strength coaches and fitness professionals have a solid understanding of anatomy, an appreciation for joint biomechanics, and the ability to assess functional strengths and weaknesses. These professionals also have the skill to integrate these components when developing a comprehensive individualized training program.

Bony Anatomy

The bony anatomy of the core includes the spine, the pelvis, and the hip joints (figure 2.1). The spinal column (also known as the vertebral column or the backbone) is made up of 33 vertebrae, along with intervertebral discs, numerous ligaments, and associated muscles. From top to bottom, the five vertebral regions are the cervical spine (7 vertebrae), the thoracic spine (12 vertebrae), the lumbar spine (5 vertebrae), the sacrum (5 fused vertebrae), and the coccyx (4 fused vertebrae) (figure 2.2). The spine connects to the pelvis via the sacrum (figure 2.3). The pelvis provides shape to the

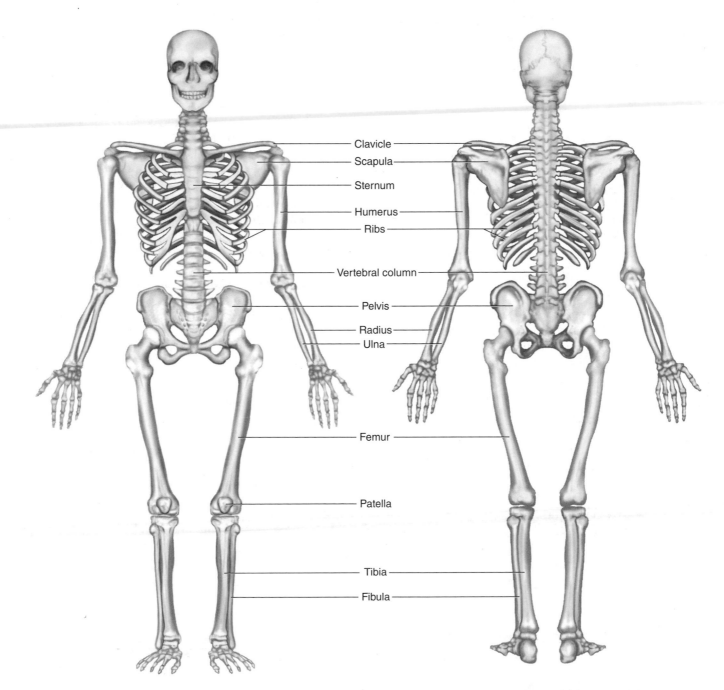

Figure 2.1 The human skeletal system. The bony anatomy of the core includes the spine, pelvis, and hip joints.

Reprinted, by permission, from NSCA, 2000, The biomechanics of resistance exercise, by E. Harman. In *Essentials of strength training and conditioning,* 2nd ed., edited by T. Baechle and R. Earle (Champaign, IL: Human Kinetics), 27.

base of the core and consists of three portions: the ilium, the ischium, and the pubis. The intersection of these three portions helps to form the acetabulum, which is the socket that the head of the thighbone (femur) fits into (figure 2.3). This is called the acetabulofemoral or hip joint.

The lumbar spine (along with the sacrum and coccyx) provides structure to the posterior and inferior parts of the core. Although the significance of the adjacent regions within the core should never be minimized, special attention and consideration should be given to the lumbar spine. As health care professionals can attest, the lumbar spine is at risk for numerous injuries. Over 80% of all people in the United States have had or will experience at least one episode of low back pain (Trainor and Wiesel 2002; Rasmussen-Barr et al. 2003). Billions of dollars are spent each year on operative and nonoperative treatments for the low back (Young et al. 1997; Luo et al. 2004; Katz 2006).

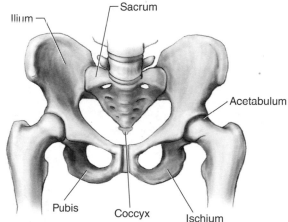

Figure 2.3 The sacrum and pelvis.

Reprinted, by permission, from R. Gotlin, 2008, *Sport injuries guidebook* (Champaign, IL: Human Kinetics), 188.

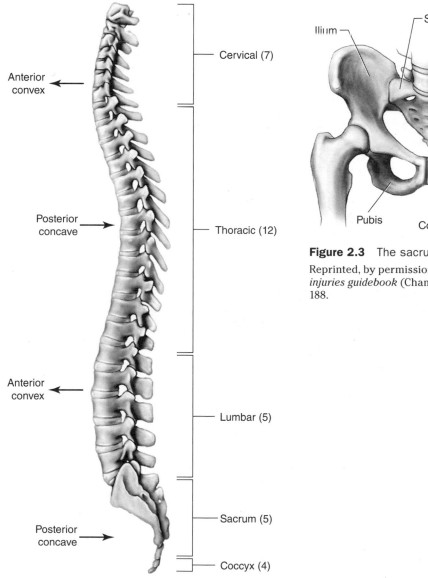

Figure 2.2 The spinal column, showing the five vertebral regions.

Reprinted from R. Behnke, 2005, *Kinetic anatomy*, 2nd ed. (Champaign, IL: Human Kinetics), 120.

Intervertebral Discs

Intervertebral discs are located between each of the cervical, thoracic, and lumbar vertebrae. Discs are made up of three components: the nucleus pulposus, the annulus fibrosus, and the end plates (figure 2.4). The discs help to absorb shock and allow mobility between each of the vertebrae. Injuries to a disc can cause significant pain and may require surgical intervention.

Muscles of the Spine

The muscles of the spine are grouped into three levels: superficial, intermediate, and deep. Figure 2.5 shows the muscles of the spine and back. The muscles in the intermediate group (the serratus posterior, superior, and inferior) assist in respiration, but they do not contribute to core stability. Therefore, this group will not be discussed here.

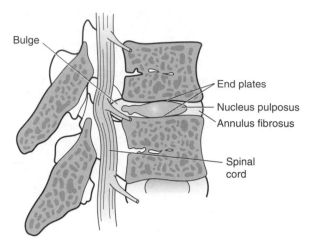

Figure 2.4 Intervertebral discs. The bulge shows one possible type of disc injury.

Reprinted, by permission, from S. Shultz, P. Houglum, and D. Perrin, 2009, *Examinations of musculoskeletal injuries,* 3rd ed. (Champaign, IL: Human Kinetics), 200.

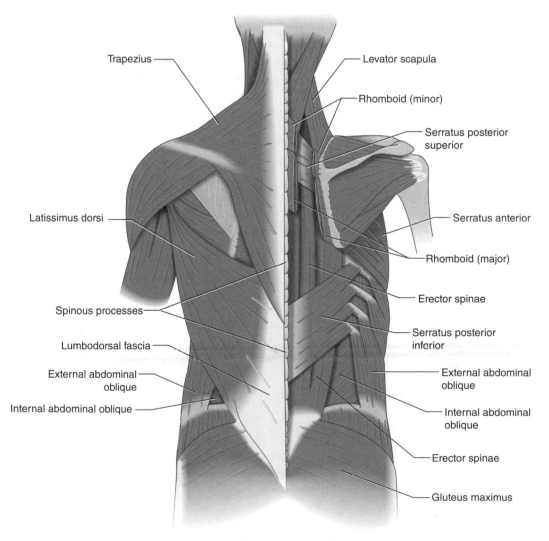

Figure 2.5 Muscles of the spine and back.

Superficial Level

The superficial muscles include the trapezius, latissimus dorsi, rhomboids (major and minor), levator scapula, and serratus anterior (figure 2.6). These superficial back muscles stabilize the scapula (shoulder blade) and assist other muscles to allow movement of the arms. Two of these muscles—the trapezius and the latissimus dorsi—contribute to core stability (see table 2.1, p. 14).

Trapezius

The trapezius, a large superficial muscle shaped like a diamond, extends from the head, runs laterally to the shoulders, and inserts near the low back (see figure 2.6). It originates on the external occipital protuberance, the ligamentum nuchae, the superior nuchal line, and the spinous processes of the C7 (cervical) to T12 (thoracic) vertebrae. The trapezius also has attachments on the lateral portion of the clavicle, the acromion, and the scapular spine.

The trapezius is divided into three sections: the superior, middle, and inferior regions. Fiber orientation dictates function (figure 2.6). The trapezius acts to elevate (superior fibers), retract (middle fibers), and depress (inferior fibers) the scapula. The superior and inferior fibers act in combination with the serratus anterior muscle to upwardly rotate the scapula, as shown in figure 2.7. The upper trapezius also assists in cervical (neck) extension, rotation of the head to the opposite side, and lateral flexion to the same side.

The trapezius appears to have a role in functional spine movements. During upper extremity functions, contraction of the trapezius will cause movement of the cervical or thoracic spinal segments. For example, contraction of the left trapezius will rotate the spinous process toward the left and the vertebral body toward the right (Neumann 2002).

The trapezius can be prone to dysfunction, posing a significant challenge for personal trainers and rehabilitation professionals. In individuals who suffer from back or shoulder pain, it is common to find **trigger points** (i.e., painful points) throughout the trapezius. When touched, a trigger point feels like a tight (taut) band. There may be pain at the site of a trigger point. The pain can also be spread (referred) to other locations. Trigger points may also limit a client's range of motion and decrease his

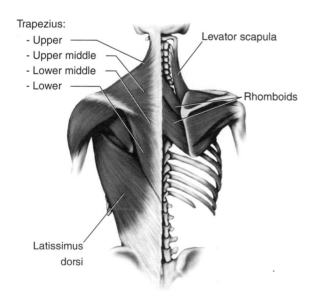

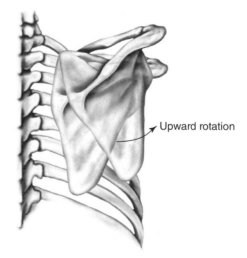

Figure 2.6 Superficial muscles of the back.

Reprinted from R. Behnke, 2005, *Kinetic anatomy*, 2nd ed. (Champaign, IL: Human Kinetics), 47.

Figure 2.7 Upward rotation of the scapula.

Reprinted, by permission, from W. Whiting and S. Rugg, 2005, *Dynatomy* (Champaign, IL: Human Kinetics), 59.

strength (Travell and Simons 1983). Even without the presence of trigger points, muscular imbalances are frequently found in the trapezius. Many clients or patients will have adequate strength in the upper trapezius while lacking functional strength in the middle or lower trapezius. Clients who have a muscular imbalance will demonstrate an upper trapezius dominance or compensation pattern with most upper extremity movements. This may be observed when a client demonstrates excessive muscular activity from the upper trapezius (e.g. shrugging during a shoulder lateral raise or during the seated rowing exercise). Also, a lack of flexibility in this muscle may contribute to or be the result of a kyphotic postural deviation (see chapter 4).

Latissimus dorsi

The latissimus dorsi originates on the spinous processes of the lower 6 thoracic vertebrae, the thoracolumbar fascia, the iliac crest, and ribs 9 through 12 (figure 2.6). The tendon of this muscle inserts in the intertubercular groove of the humerus (upper arm). The latissimus dorsi assists in extending, adducting, and internally rotating the upper arm bone. The lat pull-down machine is typically used to train this muscle.

The latissimus dorsi also serves a role in core stabilization (McGill 2002; Neumann 2002). That latissimus dorsi extends as the lumbodorsal fascia attaching to the lumbar spine. Because of this relationship, the latissimus dorsi may contribute to lumbar extension and core stabilization.

Table 2.1 Selected Superficial Muscles of the Back and Their Functional Actions on the Core

Muscles	Origins	Insertions	Functional actions
Trapezius	External occipital protuberance, ligamentum nuchae, superior nuchal line, and spinous processes of C7-T12 vertebrae	Lateral one-third of the clavicle, the acromion, and the scapular spine	Assists with scapular movement and stabilization; creates a rotatory force on the cervical and thoracic spine (Neumann 2002)
Latissimus dorsi	Spinous processes of T7-T12 vertebrae, the thoracolumbar fascia, the iliac crest, and ribs 9-12	Intertubercular groove of the humerus	Extends, adducts, and internally rotates the arm; may contribute to lumbar extension (McGill 2002)

Deep Level

The deep muscles of the back are further divided into three layers: the superficial layer, the intermediate layer, and the deep layer. The muscles of the erector spinae make up the superficial layer of deep muscles. This group of muscles have the longest muscle fiber lengths of the three layers; each layer is shorter than the previous one. The intermediate layer (also known as the transversospinalis group) is composed of the semispinalis, the multifidi, and the rotators. The deepest layer, the short segmental group, consists of two muscles: the interspinalis and the intertransversarii.

Erector spinae

The erector spinae is a large group of muscles spanning the entire length of the back (figure 2.8a, p. 16). This group consists of three muscles (presented here in order from medial to lateral): the spinalis (closest to the spine), the longissimus, and the iliocostalis (farthest from the spine) (see table 2.2, p. 15). These three muscles are each subdivided by anatomical region. They function to extend and laterally flex the trunk. They are also contributors to overall spine stability. For example, the erector spinae muscles provide a significant contribution to overall stability when a person is performing an exercise such as the back bridge (McGill 2002).

Table 2.2 Erector Spinae Muscles and Their Functional Actions on the Core

Muscles	Origins	Insertions	Functional actions
Spinalis	Spinous processes of lower thoracic and upper lumbar vertebrae	Spinous processes of cervical and upper thoracic vertebrae	Extension of the vertebral column
Longissimus	Transverse processes of cervical, thoracic, and lumbar vertebrae	Transverse processes of cervical and thoracic vertebrae and the ribs	Extension and side bending of the vertebral column
Iliocostalis	The iliac crests and ribs 3-12	Rib angles and the transverse processes of cervical spine	Extension and side bending of the vertebral column

Transversospinalis muscle group

The transversospinalis muscle group is the intermediate section of the deep muscle layer of the back. The three layers in this group are the semispinalis (superficial level), the multifidi (intermediate level), and the rotators (deep level). These muscles originate on a transverse process (bilaterally) of a vertebra, and they insert on the spinous process (bilaterally) of a superior vertebra (one to six levels higher depending on the muscle).

The semispinalis muscle group is subdivided into three sections: thoracis, cervicis, and capitis. These muscles are generally long compared to the other transversospinalis muscles, traversing six to eight vertebral segments (table 2.3). However, their primary influence on core stability is limited to extension of the thoracic spine.

The multifidi originate on a transverse process two to four vertebrae below the attachment site at the proximal spinous process (figure 2.8b, p. 16). Patients who have a history of low back pain have been shown to demonstrate the following in their multifidi: less concentric muscle activity, significantly less endurance capacity, and changes in composition and size (Richardson et al. 1999). The multifidi (along with the transversus abdominis) have received significant attention as key contributors to core stabilization (for more information, see the discussion of the transversus abdominis later in this chapter).

The rotators, the deepest of the three transversospinalis groups, are shorter in length compared to the other two. Experts disagree about the exact function of the rotators. Some suggest that the rotators serve to rotate the spine, while others suggest that these muscles do not rotate the spine but instead serve as a position sensor (McGill 2002).

Table 2.3 Muscles of the Transversospinalis Group and Their Functional Actions on the Core

Muscles	Origins	Insertions	Functional actions
Semispinalis	Transverse processes of the lower cervical vertebrae and each thoracic vertebra	Spinous processes (six to eight levels above the associated origin site) of the cervical spine and T1-T4 vertebrae; occipital bone	Extension and lateral flexion of the vertebral column
Multifidi	Sacrum, lumbar and sacral ligaments, iliac crest, erector spinae, and transverse processes	Spinous processes (two to four levels above the associated origin site)	Extension and lateral flexion of the vertebral column; lumbar stabilization
Rotators	Transverse processes in the thoracic spine	Spinous processes in the thoracic spine (one to two levels above the associated origin site)	Proprioception

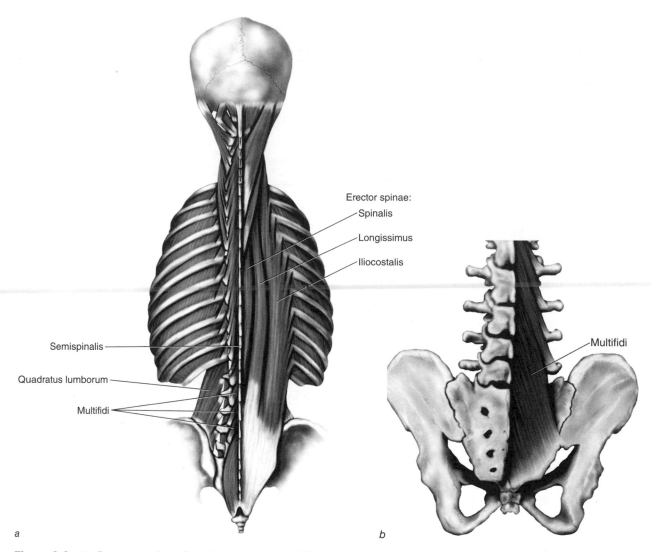

Erector spinae:
Spinalis
Longissimus
Iliocostalis

Semispinalis
Quadratus lumborum
Multifidi

Multifidi

a

b

Figure 2.8 *(a)* Deep muscles of the back and *(b)* multifidi.

Part a, reprinted from R. Behnke, 2005, *Kinetic anatomy*, 2nd ed. (Champaign, IL: Human Kinetics), 134. Part b reprinted, by permission, from J. DeWerd, 2010, *Managing low back problems* (Champaign, IL: Human Kinetics), 12.

Short segmental group

This group is the deepest layer of muscle in the back. The short segmental group consists of the intertransversarii and the interspinalis muscles. The intertransversarii muscles attach to adjacent transverse processes. The interspinalis muscles attach between adjacent spinous processes. The intertransversarii muscles contract to laterally flex the spine, and the interspinalis muscles contract to extend the spine. Together these muscles provide lumbar stabilization.

Abdomen

When someone says "abs," the first thing that comes to mind for many people is the six-pack. For many, including fitness clients, the abdomen has been marginalized to include just one muscle—the rectus abdominis. However, the abdominal region is composed of several key muscles that contribute to core function. The abdomen is the region lying between the proximal chest and the distal pelvis. This region is served by several muscles that contribute to spine stability in a variety of postures, providing the ability to flex, side bend, and rotate the trunk. These muscles also serve to protect the abdominal organs. Four muscles provide shape and movement to the anterior abdominal wall (figure 2.9). Three of these muscles are described as flat muscles (the obliques and the transversus abdominis), and one is described as being straplike (the rectus abdominis).

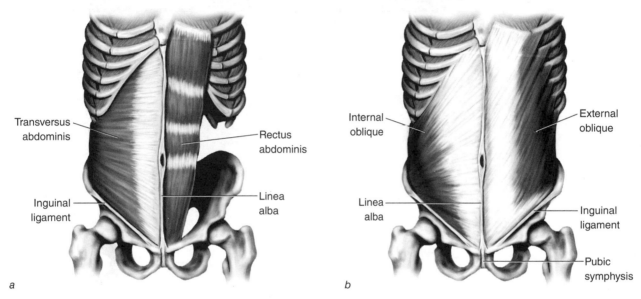

Figure 2.9 The abdominal muscles, *(a)* rectus abdominis and transversus abdominis, *(b)* obliques.
Reprinted from R. Behnke, 2005, *Kinetic anatomy*, 2nd ed. (Champaign, IL: Human Kinetics), 132.

Rectus Abdominis

The rectus abdominis (RA)—the muscle made famous in movies and television—provides both core stability and trunk mobility (figure 2.9). The RA is a trunk flexor. This muscle arises from the xiphoid process and adjacent costal cartilages, and it attaches distally into the pubic bone at the crest and symphysis. The RA muscle is trained when an individual performs an exercise such as the crunch.

Transversus Abdominis

The transversus abdominis (TA) is the deepest of the three flat abdominal muscles. The TA originates from the lower six costal cartilages, the thoracolumbar fascia, and the iliac crest; this muscle attaches medially at the linea alba (figure 2.9). The TA is reported to play a significant role in core stabilization, especially during rehabilitation (Richardson et al. 1999).

Obliques

The external and internal oblique muscles rotate and side bend the trunk. These muscles also contribute to spinal stability.

The external oblique is the most superficial muscle of the three flat abdominal muscles (the external oblique, internal oblique, and transversus abdominis). The external oblique arises from the front lateral portion of the lower seven ribs, and it inserts into the linea alba, the pubic tubercle, and the anterior portion of the iliac crest (figure 2.9). Acting alone, the external oblique can flex the trunk, side bend the torso toward the same side (i.e., the side of the contracting muscle), and rotate the trunk toward the opposite side.

The internal oblique originates from the thoracolumbar fascia, the inguinal ligament, and the anterior iliac crest. The internal oblique also functions to provide spine stability, and it flexes and rotates the trunk toward the same side (table 2.4).

Table 2.4   Muscles of the Abdominal Wall and Their Functional Actions on the Core

Muscles	Origins	Insertions	Functional actions
Rectus abdominis	Xiphoid process and adjacent costal cartilages (of ribs 5-7)	Pubic bone at the crest and symphysis	Flexes the trunk
Transversus abdominis	Thoracolumbar fascia, inguinal ligament, iliac crest, and ribs 6-12	Linea alba and pubic crest	Provides core stabilization; compresses abdominal wall
External oblique	Anterolateral (front and lateral) portion of the lower 7 ribs	Linea alba, pubic tubercle, and anterior portion of the iliac crest	Flexes the trunk; side bends the torso toward the same side (side of the contracting muscle); rotates the trunk toward the opposite side
Internal oblique	Thoracolumbar fascia, inguinal ligament, and anterior iliac crest	Linea alba and lower 4 ribs	Provides spine stability; flexes and rotates the trunk toward the same side

Pelvis and Hips

The muscles of the pelvis and hips help to stabilize the trunk, generate force, and transfer forces from the lower body to the upper body or vice versa. For example, the baseball pitcher who cannot generate powerful hip extension during the pitching motion may not be able to maximize his pitching velocity.

The hip also appears to play a significant role in proximal stabilization and control of lower extremity biomechanics. Retrospective investigations have found that injured runners are significantly weaker on their injured side when compared with their non-injured (or contralateral) leg (Niemuth et al. 2005). The muscles of the pelvis and hips that contribute to core stabilization are shown in figure 2.10.

Iliacus and Psoas Major

The iliacus and psoas major muscles are frequently called the iliopsoas in both training and clinical settings. The iliacus arises from the sacrum and iliac fossa. The psoas major (figure 2.10b) arises from the transverse processes of vertebrae T12 to L5 and the associated intervertebral discs. Both muscles combine near the inguinal ligament, forming a single tendon and inserting into the lesser trochanter on the femur. These two large muscles are traditionally viewed as hip flexors.

Gluteus Maximus

The largest of the gluteal muscles, the gluteus maximus, originates from the posterior aspect of the pelvis, the sacrum, the coccyx, and the sacrotuberous ligament. This muscle inserts into the gluteal tuberosity and the fascia lata at the iliotibial band (figure 2.10a). The muscle acts to extend and externally rotate the hip joint.

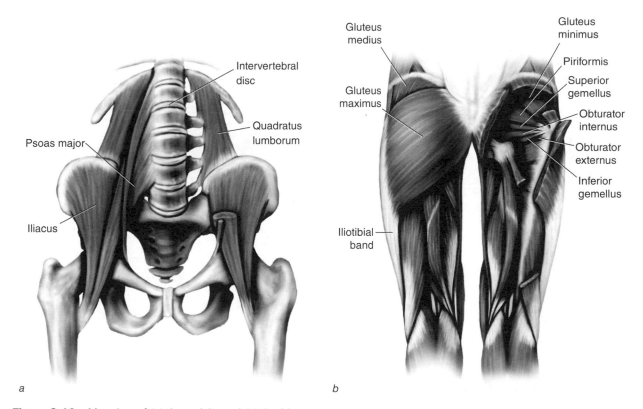

Figure 2.10   Muscles of (a) the pelvis and (b) the hips.

Reprinted from R. Behnke, 2005, *Kinetic anatomy*, 2nd ed. (Champaign, IL: Human Kinetics), 180, 178.

Gluteus Medius

The gluteus medius originates on the lateral side of the ilium, and it inserts into the greater trochanter of the femur (figure 2.10a). The gluteus medius abducts and rotates the hip. The anterior fibers of the muscle rotate the hip internally, whereas the posterior fibers externally rotate the hip.

Gluteus Minimus

The gluteus minimus, which lies deeper than the gluteus medius, originates on the lateral ilium and inserts on the anterior portion of the greater trochanter. The gluteus minimus abducts and internally rotates the hip (figure 2.10a).

Tensor Fasciae Latae

The tensor fasciae latae (TFL) arises from the upper portion of the anterior iliac spine, the iliac crest, and the fascia lata. The TFL inserts into the iliotibial band (figure 2.11). The tensor fasciae latae is better known for its long tendinous extension, the iliotibial band (IT band). The TFL provides stability to the hip and knee joint by creating tension within the IT band. Additionally, the TFL can abduct the thigh and assist with internal rotation of the hip. The iliotibial band is at risk of injury in some runners because of repetitive flexion and extension at the knee (Khaund and Flynn 2005).

Piriformis

The piriformis muscle originates from the sacrum and ilium, and it attaches to the greater trochanter of the femur (figure 2.12). This muscle functions to externally

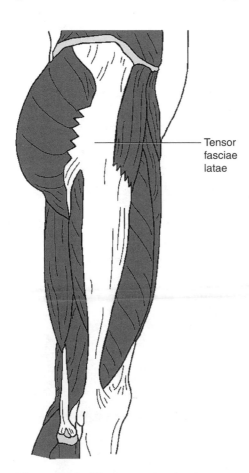

Tensor fasciae latae

Figure 2.11 The tensor fasciae latae.

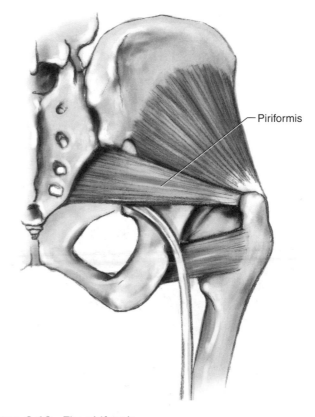

Piriformis

Figure 2.12 The piriformis.
Reprinted, by permission, from B. McAtee and J. Charland, 2007, *Facilitated stretching,* 3rd ed. (Champaign, IL: Human Kinetics), 44.

rotate and abduct the leg when the hip is in a flexed position. Trainers who provide postrehab training services may work with clients who may be experiencing tightness or weakness in the piriformis.

Inferior Gemellus

The inferior gemellus is a smaller muscle located on the posterior portion of the pelvis. This muscle originates from the posterior portion of the ischial tuberosity and attaches to the greater trochanter (figure 2.10a). When this muscle is activated, it externally rotates the thigh and helps to abduct a flexed thigh.

Obturator Externus

Arising from the outer surface of the obturator membrane and the obturator foramen, the obturator externus muscle attaches to the posterior middle surface of the greater trochanter (figure 2.10a). The obturator externus helps to externally rotate and adduct the thigh.

Obturator Internus

The obturator internus originates from the inner surface of the obturator membrane and the obturator foramen. This muscle attaches to the medial side of the greater trochanter (figure 2.10a). It helps to externally rotate and abduct the thigh.

Superior Gemellus

The superior gemellus originates from the spine of the ischium and attaches to the medial portion of the greater trochanter (figure 2.10a). This muscle externally rotates the thigh and helps to abduct the leg when the hip is flexed.

Quadratus Lumborum

The quadratus lumborum rises from the iliac crest and iliolumbar ligament on both sides of the spine, attaching to the 12th rib and the transverse processes of the L1 to L4 vertebrae (figure 2.10b). When contracting bilaterally, the quadratus lumborum functions as a lumbar extensor and stabilizer of the spine. When firing unilaterally, it flexes the trunk and it can raise the hip (table 2.5).

Table 2.5 Muscles of the Hip and Their Functional Action on the Core

Muscles	Origins	Insertions	Functional actions
Iliacus	Sacrum and iliac fossa	Lesser trochanter of the femur	Serves as a hip flexor
Psoas major	Transverse processes of vertebrae T12 to L5 and the associated intervertebral discs	Lesser trochanter of the femur	Serves as a hip flexor
Gluteus maximus	Posterior aspect of the pelvis, the sacrum, the coccyx, and the sacrotuberous ligament	Gluteal tuberosity and the fascia lata at the iliotibial band	Extends the hip; laterally rotates the thigh
Gluteus medius	Lateral side of the ilium	Greater trochanter of the femur	Abducts and rotates the hip (the anterior fibers of the muscle rotate the hip internally, whereas the posterior fibers externally rotate the hip)
Gluteus minimus	Lateral ilium	Greater trochanter (anterior portion)	Abducts and medially rotates the thigh
Tensor fasciae latae	Upper anterior iliac spine, the iliac crest, and the fascia lata	Iliotibial band	Provides stability to the hip and knee joint by creating tension within the IT band; abducts the thigh and assists with medial rotation of the hip
Piriformis	Sacrum and ilium	Greater trochanter of the femur	Laterally rotates and abducts the leg when the hip is in a flexed position
Inferior gemellus	Posterior portion of the ischial tuberosity	Greater trochanter of the femur	Laterally rotates the thigh and abducts a flexed thigh
Obturator externus	Obturator membrane and obturator foramen	Posteromedial (posterior and middle) surface of the greater trochanter	Laterally rotates and adducts the thigh
Obturator internus	Surface of the obturator membrane and the obturator foramen	Medial side of the greater trochanter	Laterally rotates and abducts the thigh
Superior gemellus	Spine of the ischium	Medial portion of the greater trochanter	Laterally rotates the thigh and helps to abduct the leg when the hip is flexed
Quadratus lumborum	Iliac crest and iliolumbar ligament on both sides of the spine	The 12th rib and the transverse processes of L1-L4 vertebrae	Functions as a lumbar extensor and stabilizer of the spine (when the muscle is contracting bilaterally); flexes the trunk and can raise the hip (when the muscle is firing unilaterally)

STRUCTURE AND FUNCTION INTEGRATION

Each client, athlete, or patient will have at least one reason for beginning a supervised exercise program. For example, a client may hire a fitness professional to design an exercise program that will reduce the risk of sustaining a back injury. Take the case of Scott, a 35-year-old longshoreman who injured his back on the job and was diagnosed by his physician with a lumbar disc injury. His physician prescribed anti-inflammatory and pain medications and restricted him to "light duty" for 4 weeks. Eventually Scott was able to return to his normal job duties. However, without proper rehabilitation or training, he may still have functional weaknesses that could potentially put him at risk for a reinjury.

In chapter 1, the following roles of core stability training were highlighted:

- To improve a client's physical fitness
- To prevent or rehabilitate an injury
- To stabilize and protect the spine from potentially injurious forces
- To enhance athletic performance by improving a client's ability to generate force and movement

To design safe and effective training programs, you need to have a working knowledge of the functional anatomy of the core. By understanding functional anatomy, you can develop an appropriate core training program based on the client's functional weaknesses and personal training goals. Would Scott, the aforementioned client, benefit from a training program? Most definitely. Scott should be considered an *industrial athlete* and should be trained accordingly. If you were designing a program for Scott, the types of exercises that you select would depend on your ability to recognize his functional limitations. You must be able to select specific flexibility and strengthening exercises that will maximize his function and maintain (or improve) his current level of health.

When designing an exercise program for a client, you need to evaluate and understand the human body in its entirety. A training program will fail if it treats body segments as individual units operating in isolation; instead, the program should address how the body functions as a whole. For example, many core rehabilitation programs include the use of isometric exercises performed in supine or prone positions. These exercises may be necessary for clients who are starting a fitness or injury rehabilitation program. However, limiting a training or rehabilitation program to these basic exercises will fail to address the dynamic functional movement patterns necessary for daily activities and sport performance. How would basic core exercises affect the functional outcomes for Scott, our hypothetical client? Most human activities involve a dynamic interaction between the regions of the body (the upper extremities, the trunk, and the lower extremities); these regions must operate synergistically to create functional movement patterns.

The **kinetic link principle** describes how joints and muscles interact with each other during a functional movement pattern. This principle is defined as follows:

> The kinetic link principle describes how the human body can be considered as a series of interrelated links or segments. Movement of one segment affects segments both proximal and distal to the first segment. (Ellenbecker and Davies 2001, p. 19)

To illustrate this point, let's apply the kinetic link principle to the knee. The knee joint (a link) has its own unique anatomy and biomechanics (e.g., the knee is affected by the mechanics and musculature of the hip as well as that of the lower leg and ankle).

During a functional movement pattern, such as descending stairs, the biomechanics at the knee will be influenced by hip as well as foot and ankle interactions

(Ellenbecker and Davies 2001; Powers 2003). Poor hip strength may lead to **adduction** and **internal rotation** movements at the hip, causing the knee to rotate inward as the leg accepts weight during each descending step (Powers 2003). In some individuals, this less-than-optimal biomechanical interaction may contribute to the development of anterior knee pain.

Because the core is centrally located, it can affect the function of both upper and lower extremities. To appreciate the role of the core in a sport application, consider the biomechanics of the tennis serve. For an athlete to be successful at tennis, she must be both quick and agile (Roetert et al. 1997). The tennis player must have an adequate endurance capacity to sustain a high level of play throughout the competition. This athlete must also have the ability to generate and transfer forces in order to maximize racket acceleration. Failure to perform at a high level—integrating components of speed, strength, power, and endurance—may make the difference between winning a championship and losing in the first round.

The ability to synergistically integrate each segment within the kinetic chain is vital to athletic success at the highest levels. Professional tennis player Andy Roddick can overpower his competition by serving at speeds over 150 miles per hour. For any tennis player to serve at a comparable speed, the player's body segments must optimally operate in sequence. During the tennis serve, a significant portion of force development is created by the lower extremities and the trunk (Kibler 1994; Ellenbecker and Davies 2001). Figure 2.13 illustrates how a ground reaction force is created and then sequentially transferred from one segment to the next in a proximal-to-distal sequence. If Andy Roddick, or any other tennis player, attempted to activate his shoulder muscles (the distal segment) before the force contribution of the hip musculature (the proximal segment), the movement pattern would be dysfunctional, and performance would be affected.

Biomechanical dysfunction will also increase the athlete's risk of developing an overuse injury. Figures 2.14 and 2.15 highlight dysfunctional muscle activation and improper timing between sequential links in the kinetic chain (Ellenbecker and

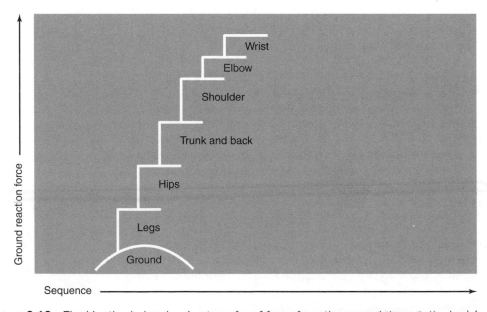

Figure 2.13 The kinetic chain, showing transfer of force from the ground through the body's segments.

Reprinted, by permission, from T. Ellenbecker and G. Davies, 2001, *Closed kinetic chain exercise* (Champaign, IL: Human Kinetics), 21; and adapted from J.L. Groppel. 1992, *High tech tennis,* 2nd ed. (Champaign, IL: Human Kinetics), 79. By permission of J.L. Groppel.

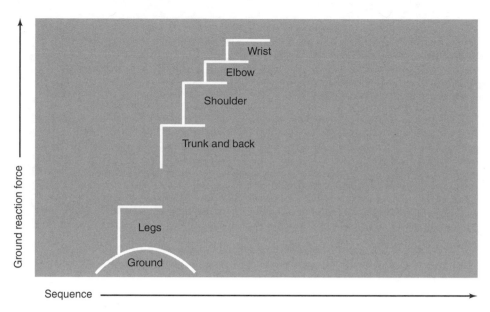

Figure 2.14   Kinetic chain, showing a dysfunctional pattern due to a missing link the in the sequence.

Reprinted, by permission, from T. Ellenbecker and G. Davies, 2001, *Closed kinetic chain exercise* (Champaign, IL: Human Kinetics), 22; and adapted from J.L. Groppel. 1992, *IIigh tech tennis,* 2nd ed. (Champaign, IL: Human Kinetics), 79. By permission of J.L. Groppel.

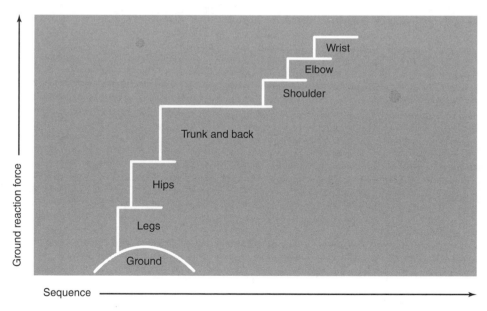

Figure 2.15   Kinetic chain, showing a dysfunctional pattern due to a delay in the trunk and back portion of the sequence.

Reprinted, by permission, from T. Ellenbecker and G. Davies, 2001, *Closed kinetic chain exercise* (Champaign, IL: Human Kinetics), 22; and adapted, from J.L. Groppel. 1992, *High tech tennis,* 2nd ed. (Champaign, IL: Human Kinetics), 79. By permission of J.L. Groppel.

Davies 2001). The tennis player who is sidelined by a shoulder or elbow injury may have sustained that injury in part because of a dysfunctional core. To reduce these types of injuries and enhance sport performance, core exercises must be included in a comprehensive training program.

SUMMARY

The core is a vital component of the kinetic chain. For sports and many functional tasks, the core is a key link in the proximal-to-distal sequencing of forces from the ground to the upper extremities. Dysfunction in the core may affect human performance and contribute to the onset of an injury.

The core is made up of more than just the muscles. Fitness professionals must understand the function of the related anatomy (e.g., joints, intervertebral discs) and how these structures interact with the musculature during human movement. These structures are at risk of injury, and special training considerations must be followed in order to reduce this risk of injury (or reinjury).

The functional anatomy of the core should create the foundation for each training program that you design. Appreciating that segments of the body operate synergistically will help you recognize when to prescribe exercises that isolate movement and when to integrate functional multijoint movements.

3

The Client Interview

The First Step in Assessing Your Client

How convenient would it be if the same training program could be prescribed to each individual who enlisted your services? Of course, if this were the case, many professionals who prescribe exercises would find themselves out of work! Although similarities may exist between individuals, you need to understand that each client, athlete, or patient is unique. The challenge is to develop an exercise (or rehabilitation) program based on the client's goals and physical presentation, the best available research evidence, and your own clinical experience and reasoning skills.

OBTAINING A HISTORY AND MEDICAL CLEARANCE

During your initial meeting with your client you should obtain their medical and exercise history. When necessary, you may ask the client to obtain medical clearance from their primary care provider prior to initiating their training program. Failing to fully assess and consider a client's pertinent medical history may put you at risk for a lawsuit if you were to prescribe unsafe or contraindicated exercises. Failing to assess the client's exercise history and fitness goals would also limit your ability to develop an optimal core training program for that individual.

The PAR-Q (form 3.1, p. 32) and client history forms (form 3.2, p. 34) will help you screen clients for any conditions that might require a physician's clearance (Shephard 1988; Thomas et al. 1992). This screening should be done before you conduct fitness tests or start the client on an exercise program. The PAR-Q screens for known disease and for medical conditions that might affect exercise (Shephard 1988; Thomas et al. 1992). It is designed to be used with individuals who are between 15 and 69 years old.

If the PAR-Q indicates that the client is apparently healthy (i.e., the client answers no to all of the PAR-Q questions), you can then proceed to reviewing the person's client history form (Shephard 1988; Thomas et al. 1992). This form will help you determine if any other conditions exist that may prohibit the client from having a fitness assessment and participating in an exercise program. The client history form also provides valuable information about the client's exercise habits and preferences as well as the client's lifestyle.

If a client answers yes to one or more of the PAR-Q questions, then the client must see a physician before you conduct any fitness tests or teach any exercises (Shephard 1988; Thomas et al. 1992). You can provide the client with a PARmed-X form, also available from the Canadian Society for Exercise Physiology, for his physician to complete (Jamnik et al. 2007). This form allows the physician to identify any restrictions on fitness testing or exercises for the client. If a client has an orthopedic condition and is currently under the care of a rehabilitation professional—such as a physical therapist, athletic trainer, or occupational therapist—you should also have the client seek permission and guidance from this professional regarding the initiation of a core training program. Once the client has returned the PARmed-X form and has given you any other pertinent medical clearance forms, you can proceed to completing your fitness assessment.

After completing your review of the client history form, you will be better prepared to begin your client interview.

INTERVIEWING YOUR CLIENT

When you take your car to an automotive shop for repairs, you expect the mechanic to ask a series of questions in order to better understand the car's "symptoms" before initiating any repairs. From that first conversation, you may gain a sense of what is wrong with the car and the estimated costs of the repairs. More important, if you believe that you have been listened to, had all of your questions answered, and been treated in a favorable manner, you are likely to have confidence in the mechanic. You may even want to refer friends and family to that particular shop. On the other hand, if the mechanic fails to listen to you, doesn't answer or acknowledge your questions, and doesn't take the time to have a dialogue with you, you are likely to take your car down the road to the competition.

Whether you develop exercise programs for healthy clients or for injured clients, you must make sure to conduct a thorough interview with each individual. During the first appointment, take as much time as necessary to interview your new client. When conducting the interview, it is important to actively listen to what the client has to say. Failing to listen to a client may affect the training program you design. In addition, failing to be attentive to your client's needs is a good way to lose that client as a customer.

The following list consists of some common questions that you should ask when collecting information from a patient or fitness client. The list provides a series of questions that are applicable for the clients of personal trainers, strength and conditioning professionals, and rehabilitation specialists. You may also want to collect additional information on an individual basis. These additional questions often arise naturally through the interview process. Rehabilitation specialists should ask additional questions that are specific to their respective profession.

■ *Why is the client seeking your services? What are the client's goals?* Your most important objective during the initial interview is to gain an understanding of why the client is seeking your services. This will enable you to develop specific training goals (in conjunction with your client). The core exercises you include in the client's or athlete's training program will be dependent on these goals.

• *Goal-setting considerations for athletes.* Some athletes may express generic training goals such as "I want to be stronger" or "I want to jump higher." Identifying these general goals can be useful. After all, who knows an athlete's limitations better than the athlete himself? However, a goal such as "I want to jump higher" is too subjective. In this situation, you need to quantify what the athlete means by "stronger" and "higher." Communicating with the coaching staff and performing a needs analysis will help you quantify the athlete's goals. For example, the "jump higher" goal can be quantified with a vertical jump test. A basketball forward who wants to jump higher in order to dunk the ball might have a quantifiable goal of training to increase his vertical jump height by 8 inches (20 cm).

• *Goal-setting considerations for injured clients or patients.* Injured clients will have the goal of decreasing their pain and improving their function. For example, a 45-year-old fledgling runner sustains a knee injury after increasing her mileage. She seeks the assistance of a rehabilitation professional to decrease her pain and to help her return to running. But effective rehabilitation goes beyond doing the obvious, such as strengthening the quadriceps. The training program for this client should address underlying core issues that may also be contributing to the client's knee pain. Thus, rehabilitation professionals must help injured clients realize that they should have additional goals besides decreasing pain and returning to their sport or daily activities.

Personal trainers and strength coaches who are working with clients postrehab (the period of time between a client's formal discharge from clinical rehabilitation and the point at which the client has reached maximal recovery) should consider asking their clients to sign a release for their rehabilitation specialist. This will allow the trainer to contact the rehabilitation specialist to learn more about the client's diagnosis and previous interventions.

• *Goal-setting considerations for clients of personal trainers.* Hiring a personal trainer is the first step for many people who want to improve their overall health and fitness. For some, the main goal might be to lose weight.

Medical and Allied Health Care Professionals Who Treat Musculoskeletal Injuries

Each year, hundreds of thousands of individuals seek medical attention for musculoskeletal injuries in the United States. For these injuries, people may get help from various types of health care professionals. The sidebar lists some of the health care professionals a client may seek out.

Medical doctor (MD)

Doctor of osteopathy (DO)

Doctor of podiatric medicine (DPM)

Physical therapist (PT)

Athletic trainer (ATC)

Physician assistant (PA)

Nurse practitioner (NP)

Occupational therapist (OT)

Chiropractor (DC)

Licensed massage therapist (LMT)

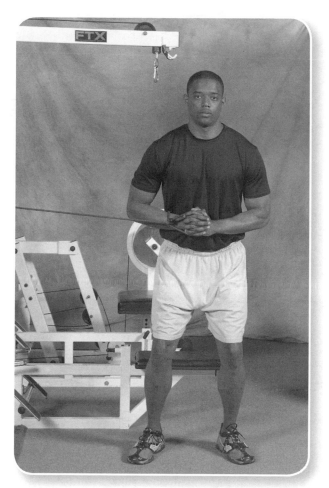

Figure 3.1   Straight-plane cable rotation exercise. To perform this exercise, the client begins in this position (as in the cable side steps exercise, p. 63) and then rotates the torso away from the machine.

Others may have a specific functional goal that they want to reach. For example, a 35-year-old male who is a recreational golfer may have a specific goal of increasing his driving distance. To help him achieve this goal, you would need to perform a core assessment on him and give him an individualized training program based on the assessment. Giving him a generic one-size-fits-all training program will not address his specific core deficits and will likely be unsuccessful in helping him meet his goal. The core exercise program you create for the golfer should be significantly different from a program designed for a client whose primary goal is weight loss. And, the core exercise program for one golfer may differ significantly from the program for another golfer.

■ *What is the client's age?* The client's age must always be considered when selecting core exercises. The approach to designing a core training program for a 65-year-old client should differ drastically from the approach used when designing a program for an 18-year-old. When training the senior client, you must note preexisting orthopedic impairments, experience with exercise training, mobility status, risk for falls, and cognitive status.

You could consider implementing a straight-plane cable rotation exercise (figure 3.1) for a 65-year-old who plays golf and tennis. On the other hand, for a 70-year-old client who has significant balance and mobility issues, a floor program that involves dynamic core exercises would be inappropriate. For this client, a more appropriate program is one that includes very basic standing exercises such as the wall lean (figure 3.2) and the straight-arm pull-down (figure 3.3).

■ *What is the client's occupation?* A job takes up a significant portion of a person's daily life. For many, their employment is dependent on how their machine (i.e., body) functions! However, the repetitive nature of many jobs contributes to a host of occupational overuse injuries (e.g., carpal tunnel syndrome, neck strain, and so on). Special clinics are devoted to the evaluation and treatment of employees who have been injured on

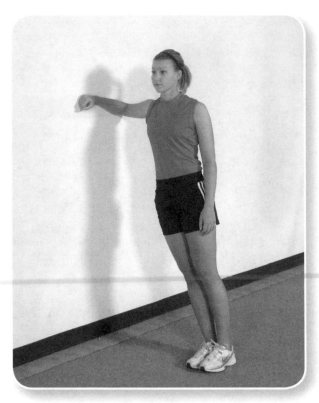

Figure 3.2 Wall lean. See page 62 for complete instructions for this exercise.

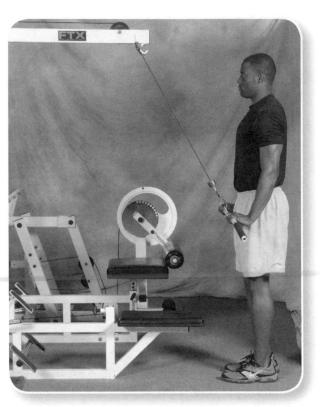

Figure 3.3 Straight-arm pull-down. See page 62 for complete instructions for this exercise.

the job. As mentioned in chapter 1, work-related injuries account for missed time from work, millions of dollars spent on health care, and for some, a permanent disability. When designing a strength training program, you should assess the client's work environment and the physical requirements of the client's job. Part of this assessment will involve asking the client questions such as the following: "Do you sit for extended periods of time?" "Do you repetitively lift heavy objects?" "Do you work at a computer? If so, are the keyboard and monitor positioned in a manner that places undue stress on your neck or wrists?" Your exercise selection should address a client's functional job requirements.

■ *Has the client participated in an exercise program in the past?* Your client's current fitness level should help guide your decisions regarding not only what exercises to initially prescribe, but also how quickly to progress the client's program. An athlete may be able to quickly progress from basic to advanced exercises. However, a sedentary individual may require additional time before advancing from one exercise stage to the next.

■ *Has the client ever experienced a low back injury or other orthopedic injury?* In your review of the client's PAR-Q and client history forms, you should identify any history of a low back injury or other orthopedic injury. If the client has had this type of injury, you should make sure the client has medical clearance to participate in a core training program. You should also ask the client to identify any previous episodes of pain in the low back or other injured area, what event caused the pain, and what factors (activities) worsen the pain. Individuals who are experiencing (or have experienced) low back pain will likely benefit from a core stability training program.

If a client has a history of back injury or pain, nonmedical fitness professionals should ask additional questions. Does the client know the name of the injury or condition that she was previously diagnosed with? Was the injury a ruptured vertebral disc or a muscle strain? Can the client describe the severity of previous or current back problems or injuries? Is the client aware of movements or exercises that aggravate the condition? How long did previous episodes of back pain last? What events have caused or brought on the back pain? What interventions have helped resolve the pain in the past?

Use the information you collect to help guide your decision making when prescribing exercises. When you design the client's core training program, you should avoid prescribing exercises that may increase the risk of reaggravating the client's back pain. For example, consider the case of a 37-year-old construction worker who sustained a lumbar disk injury at the L4-L5 level. The patient was unable to work due to the significant pain associated with this injury. He was referred by his family physician to physical therapy. After 8 weeks of physical therapy he was pain-free and his functional abilities were restored. The physical therapist instructed the patient how to lift properly at work and discharged him with a home exercise program (HEP). The patient was compliant with his HEP and was able to do all of his job requirements without pain. In order to improve his overall fitness, he sought the services of a personal trainer. During the initial appointment, the trainer had him perform the T-bar row exercise, in which a weighted bar is pulled toward the torso, with heavy weights for 3 sets of 10 repetitions. Ideally, clients maintain a neutral spine position throughout this movement; however, it is not uncommon to observe clients either excessively flexing or extending the lumbar spine during the exercise. Four hours after the session, the client experienced intense back pain and a loss of strength in his right leg. He was transferred to the emergency room to address his pain. Imaging studies revealed that he reinjured the L4-L5 lumbar disk. His orthopedic surgeon recommended surgery to perform an L4-L5 lumbar **discectomy** the next day. What went wrong? The personal trainer failed to recognize that the T-bar row exercise was potentially unsafe for this client. The T-bar row, even when performed correctly, may excessively stress the lumbar spine.

You must also consider other orthopedic injuries sustained by your clients. As with back injuries, any client who has experienced a significant injury or pain should be evaluated by a medical professional. If the client comes to you first, you should refer the client to her physician. A medical care professional such as a physical therapist, athletic trainer, or occupational therapist should assume responsibility for developing an appropriate rehabilitation program for the client's injury. However, you will likely be working with clients who have had past injuries that don't currently preclude their participation in a core training program. For these clients, you should still consider the injury and any exercises that could reinjure the area or cause a flare-up of pain. For example, the side plank is frequently included in core training programs. This is an ideal exercise for activating the transversus abdominis, the obliques, and the quadratus lumborum (McGill 2002). However, the side plank would not be an appropriate exercise for a client who has a history of shoulder pain.

SUMMARY

Interviewing your client is the crucial first step in developing a professional relationship. You must always conduct a client interview before initiating a training or rehabilitation program. Failing to listen to and learn from your client will adversely affect your program design. It might also cost you clientele.

During the interview process, you should be able to identify the client's personal fitness goals. You should also identify the client's current fitness habits, find out about the client's previous or current medical diagnoses, and gain an understanding of how the client's unique attributes might influence program design. Each of these factors will assist you as you develop a program catered for that individual. Remember, a generic (one-size-fits-all) core program will fail to meet the functional needs of most clients. Once the client interview process has been completed you will conduct a functional evaluation. This evaluation will enable you to identify the client's functional strengths and limitations.

Physical Activity Readiness
Questionnaire - PAR-Q
(revised 2002)

PAR-Q & YOU

(A Questionnaire for People Aged 15 to 69)

Regular physical activity is fun and healthy, and increasingly more people are starting to become more active every day. Being more active is very safe for most people. However, some people should check with their doctor before they start becoming much more physically active.

If you are planning to become much more physically active than you are now, start by answering the seven questions in the box below. If you are between the ages of 15 and 69, the PAR-Q will tell you if you should check with your doctor before you start. If you are over 69 years of age, and you are not used to being very active, check with your doctor.

Common sense is your best guide when you answer these questions. Please read the questions carefully and answer each one honestly: check YES or NO.

YES	NO		
☐	☐	1.	Has your doctor ever said that you have a heart condition <u>and</u> that you should only do physical activity recommended by a doctor?
☐	☐	2.	Do you feel pain in your chest when you do physical activity?
☐	☐	3.	In the past month, have you had chest pain when you were not doing physical activity?
☐	☐	4.	Do you lose your balance because of dizziness or do you ever lose consciousness?
☐	☐	5.	Do you have a bone or joint problem (for example, back, knee or hip) that could be made worse by a change in your physical activity?
☐	☐	6.	Is your doctor currently prescribing drugs (for example, water pills) for your blood pressure or heart condition?
☐	☐	7.	Do you know of <u>any other reason</u> why you should not do physical activity?

If

you

answered

YES to one or more questions

Talk with your doctor by phone or in person BEFORE you start becoming much more physically active or BEFORE you have a fitness appraisal. Tell your doctor about the PAR-Q and which questions you answered YES.

- You may be able to do any activity you want — as long as you start slowly and build up gradually. Or, you may need to restrict your activities to those which are safe for you. Talk with your doctor about the kinds of activities you wish to participate in and follow his/her advice.
- Find out which community programs are safe and helpful for you.

NO to all questions

If you answered NO honestly to <u>all</u> PAR-Q questions, you can be reasonably sure that you can:
- start becoming much more physically active — begin slowly and build up gradually. This is the safest and easiest way to go.
- take part in a fitness appraisal — this is an excellent way to determine your basic fitness so that you can plan the best way for you to live actively. It is also highly recommended that you have your blood pressure evaluated. If your reading is over 144/94, talk with your doctor before you start becoming much more physically active.

DELAY BECOMING MUCH MORE ACTIVE:
- if you are not feeling well because of a temporary illness such as a cold or a fever — wait until you feel better; or
- if you are or may be pregnant — talk to your doctor before you start becoming more active.

PLEASE NOTE: If your health changes so that you then answer YES to any of the above questions, tell your fitness or health professional. Ask whether you should change your physical activity plan.

Informed Use of the PAR-Q: The Canadian Society for Exercise Physiology, Health Canada, and their agents assume no liability for persons who undertake physical activity, and if in doubt after completing this questionnaire, consult your doctor prior to physical activity.

No changes permitted. You are encouraged to photocopy the PAR-Q but only if you use the entire form.

NOTE: If the PAR-Q is being given to a person before he or she participates in a physical activity program or a fitness appraisal, this section may be used for legal or administrative purposes.

"I have read, understood and completed this questionnaire. Any questions I had were answered to my full satisfaction."

NAME _____

SIGNATURE _____ DATE _____

SIGNATURE OF PARENT _____ WITNESS _____
or GUARDIAN (for participants under the age of majority)

Note: This physical activity clearance is valid for a maximum of 12 months from the date it is completed and becomes invalid if your condition changes so that you would answer YES to any of the seven questions.

CSEP
SCPE © Canadian Society for Exercise Physiology   Supported by: ▮◆▮ Health   Santé
                                                                     Canada Canada   continued on other side...

Form 3.1 PAR-Q questionnaire. A form like this can be a first step when screening clients for medical conditions that might affect exercise.

From Human Kinetics, 2010, *Core Assessment and Training* (Champaign, IL: Human Kinetics).

Source: *Physical Activity Readiness Questionnaire (PAR-Q)* © 2002. Used with permission from the Canadian Society for Exercise Physiology www.csep.ca.

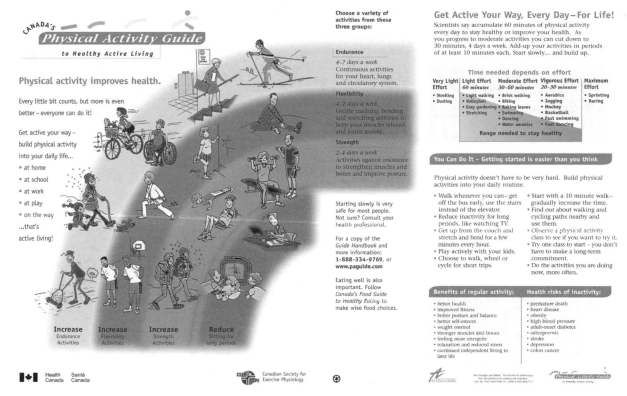

Source: *Canada's Physical Activity Guide to Healthy Active Living*, Health Canada, 1998 http://www.hc-sc.gc.ca/hppb/paguide/pdf/guideEng.pdf

© Reproduced with permission from the Minister of Public Works and Government Services Canada, 2002.

FITNESS AND HEALTH PROFESSIONALS MAY BE INTERESTED IN THE INFORMATION BELOW:

The following companion forms are available for doctors' use by contacting the Canadian Society for Exercise Physiology (address below):

The **Physical Activity Readiness Medical Examination (PARmed-X)** – to be used by doctors with people who answer YES to one or more questions on the PAR-Q.

The **Physical Activity Readiness Medical Examination for Pregnancy (PARmed-X for Pregnancy)** – to be used by doctors with pregnant patients who wish to become more active.

References:

Arraix, G.A., Wigle, D.T., Mao, Y. (1992). Risk Assessment of Physical Activity and Physical Fitness in the Canada Health Survey
Follow-Up Study. **J. Clin. Epidemiol.** 45:4 419-428.

Mottola, M., Wolfe, L.A. (1994). Active Living and Pregnancy, In: A. Quinney, L. Gauvin, T. Wall (eds.), **Toward Active Living: Proceedings of the International Conference on Physical Activity, Fitness and Health**. Champaign, IL: Human Kinetics.

PAR-Q Validation Report, British Columbia Ministry of Health, 1978.

Thomas, S., Reading, J., Shephard, R.J. (1992). Revision of the Physical Activity Readiness Questionnaire (PAR-Q). **Can. J. Spt. Sci.** 17:4 338-345.

To order multiple printed copies of the PAR-Q, please contact the:

Canadian Society for Exercise Physiology
202-185 Somerset Street West
Ottawa, ON K2P 0J2
Tel. 1-877-651-3755 • FAX (613) 234-3565
Online: www.csep.ca

The original PAR-Q was developed by the British Columbia Ministry of Health. It has been revised by an Expert Advisory Committee of the Canadian Society for Exercise Physiology chaired by Dr. N. Gledhill (2002).

Disponible en français sous le titre «Questionnaire sur l'aptitude à l'activité physique - Q-AAP (revisé 2002)».

  © Canadian Society for Exercise Physiology   Supported by: Health Canada Santé Canada

---

Form 3.1 *(continued)*

From Human Kinetics, 2010, *Core Assessment and Training* (Champaign, IL: Human Kinetics).

Source: *Physical Activity Readiness Questionnaire (PAR-Q)* © 2002. Used with permission from the Canadian Society for Exercise Physiology www.csep.ca.

Sample Client Information

Name: _____

Address: _____

Home Phone: _____ Work Phone: _____

Date of Birth: _____ Occupation: _____

Height (cm): _____ Weight (kg): _____

BMI: _____ [BMI = wt (kg)/ht (m)2]

Blood pressure: Systolic _____ mmHg _____ Diastolic _____ mmHg

Pulse: _____ bpm

Please mark each statement that is true.

_____ You are a man over the age of 45 years.

_____ You are a woman over the age of 55 years.

_____ You are physically inactive (active less than 30 minutes 3 times a week).

_____ You are overweight (20 lb [9 kg] or more, or BMI over 30).

_____ You presently smoke or have quit within the past 6 months.

_____ You have high blood pressure or take blood pressure medication.

_____ Systolic blood pressure over 140mmHg

_____ Diastolic blood pressure over 90 mmHg

_____ You have been told you have high cholesterol.

_____ Your father or brother had a heart attack or heart surgery before the age of 55.

_____ Your mother or sister had a heart attack or heart surgery before the age of 65.

Exercise habits

_____ Intensive occupational and recreational exertion

_____ Moderate occupational and recreational exertion

_____ Sedentary work and intense recreational exertion

_____ Sedentary work and moderate recreational exertion

_____ Sedentary work and light recreational exertion

_____ Complete lack of occupational or recreational exertion

Any reason why you can't exercise regularly? _____

Form 3.2 If the PAR-Q indicates that the client is apparently healthy, a form like this one will help you determine if any other relevant conditions exist and provide information about the client's exercise habits and lifestyle.

From Human Kinetics, 2010, *Core Assessment and Training* (Champaign, IL: Human Kinetics).

Reprinted, by permission, from Can-Fit-Pro, 2008, *Foundations of professional personal training* (Champaign, IL: Human Kinetics), 104-106.

What exercises do you enjoy or have you enjoyed in the past?

1. _____

2. _____

3. _____

Existing medical conditions

Please check the appropriate conditions.

____ Anemia	____ Epilepsy	____ Pregnancy
____ Arthritis	____ Heart condition	____ Thyroid problems
____ Asthma	____ Hernia	____ Ulcer
____ Cholesterol	____ Obesity	____ Other: _____
____ Diabetes		

Medications

Are you currently taking any medications? ____ Yes ____ No

If yes, please list the medication and for what condition.

Medication: _____ Condition: _____

Medication: _____ Condition: _____

Medication: _____ Condition: _____

Medication: _____ Condition: _____

Allergies

Do you have any allergies? ____ Yes ____ No

If yes, please list and indicate if medication is required.

Allergy: _____ Medication required: _____

Allergy: _____ Medication required: _____

Injuries

Do you have pain in, or have you injured any of the following areas?

____ Neck	____ Shoulder: R / L	____ Hip: R / L
____ Upper back	____ Elbow: R / L	____ Knee: R / L
____ Lower back	____ Wrist: R / L	____ Ankle R / L

Please explain: _____

_____

_____

(continued)

Form 3.2 *(continued)*

From Human Kinetics, 2010, *Core Assessment and Training* (Champaign, IL: Human Kinetics).

Reprinted, by permission, from Can-Fit-Pro, 2008, *Foundations of professional personal training* (Champaign, IL: Human Kinetics), 104-106.

Contact in Case of Emergency

Name: _____

Phone number: _____

Relation: _____

Family physician

Name: _____

City: _____

Phone number: _____

Lifestyle

	Always	Sometimes	Rarely
I get 7-8 hours of sleep per night	____	____	____
I am physically active 3 times a week	____	____	____
I have regular medical checkups	____	____	____
I eat 3-5 servings of vegetables daily	____	____	____
I eat 2-4 servings of fruit daily	____	____	____
I eat 6-10 servings of grains and cereals daily	____	____	____
I eat 2-3 servings of meats and nuts daily	____	____	____
I make a conscious effort to eat healthy	____	____	____
I follow a strict diet	____	____	____
I have no stress in my life	____	____	____
I am a very happy person	____	____	____
I am highly motivated	____	____	____

Personal Trainer

By signing this form, I certify that I have asked for and understand the pertinent information required for me to make an informed decision.

Signature: _____ Date: _____

Client

By signing this form, I certify that I have fully disclosed all pertinent information in an honest and truthful manner.

Signature: _____ Date: _____

Form 3.2 *(continued)*

From Human Kinetics, 2010, *Core Assessment and Training* (Champaign, IL: Human Kinetics).

Reprinted, by permission, from Can-Fit-Pro, 2008, *Foundations of professional personal training* (Champaign, IL: Human Kinetics), 104-106.

4
Physical Assessment and Functional Testing

As discussed in the previous chapter, you should conduct an initial interview with each client to gather information regarding the client's health and fitness status. However, the training program you design will be incomplete if you rely solely on this information. You must also conduct physical assessments and functional tests to assess the client's current physical status. This will enable you to identify a baseline for the functional level of the client's core. You can then combine the findings from the client's physical assessment with the information obtained during the interview to help guide your program design.

DESCRIPTIONS OF CORE PHYSICAL ASSESSMENT

Many assessment tools can be used to help determine a client's functional level. The challenge is to choose a series of tests that will maximize your understanding of the client's functional status and that will also be within the physical and financial parameters of your setting. For example, individuals at a university hospital may have access to expensive isokinetic testing machines or balance training devices. However, strength coaches employed in the high school setting may be limited to the available gym equipment and court space. Regardless of your setting, you should be able to conduct each of the tests presented in this chapter.

Compared to testing other regions of the body, testing the core has proven to be a bit challenging. Isokinetic testing, for example, can provide objective data regarding a client's strength at various speeds. However, the design of most isokinetic machines only allows testing of the upper and lower extremities. On the other hand, a **functional test** can provide valuable information regarding the client's baseline functional status. A functional test differs from a traditional manual muscle test in that it tests strength in a functional movement pattern. As a result, some additional analysis may be necessary to interpret the findings. Unfortunately, research regarding the reliability and validity of some of these tests is often lacking.

When assessing a client's baseline status, a fitness professional should use tests that have been scientifically proven to be both **valid** and **reliable.** A test is considered valid when it measures what it is intended to measure. A test is reliable if it is shown to consistently provide the same results when it is repeated (Portney and Watkins 1999; Jewell 2008). Some functional tests have yet to be scientifically scrutinized for validity and reliability. This doesn't mean that these tests lack relevance. They can still provide valuable information to help guide exercise prescription and program design.

The following sections identify a specific sequence of tests that can be used for functionally testing the core. The testing begins with the client in a standing position, and it progresses to tests with the client in various positions on a table or mat. The order of the tests is designed to minimize the number of positional changes experienced during the testing sequence (Plastaras et al 2005).

STANDING EVALUATION

Your initial assessment of each client should begin with the client in a standing position. You can then observe the client's posture, assess active range of motion (AROM), and conduct standing functional tests.

Assessing Posture

For many people, the word *posture* evokes memories of being told to sit up or stand up straight. As if that weren't enough, when people sustain a musculoskeletal injury of the neck or back, they are often reminded by their health care providers of the benefits of proper posture.

Why is proper posture important for clients and patients? Why do health care professionals place so much value on good posture? Take a look around. How many people maintain proper sitting posture at their work space for more than 30 minutes? How about for 1 minute? For many, the occupations of life (work, hobbies, and so on) tend to limit the variety of their movement. Individuals end up confining themselves to one or two positions for prolonged periods. After a while, the body begins to adapt (tighten) in response to those positions.

Maintaining proper posture is believed to help decrease the abnormal joint loading that may contribute to arthritic changes over time. Proper posture is also purported to help decrease or eliminate joint and muscular pain. Although few studies have been done to support these claims, many people have experienced relief of aches or muscle soreness by repositioning their body from one posture to another.

Recognizing poor posture is a lot easier than defining or quantifying ideal posture. Basically, ideal posture is when a person is able to maintain a skeletal position that places the least amount of strain on the joints, muscles, and ligaments.

Plumb Line Test

Objective: To identify postural deviations

Instructions:

1. Make sure the client is properly dressed; the client's clothing should allow you to easily observe the entire spine. Have male clients take their shirts off. Have female clients wear a sports bra.

2. Hang a plumb line from the ceiling or from the top of a squat rack.

3. When you are viewing the client from the side, the line should pass just behind the client's ear (through the mastoid process of the temporal bone), in front of the sacrum, behind the hip joint, and to the front of both the knee and ankle joints (see figure 4.1). The line should also fall to the *concave* side of each of the spine's curves.

4. In addition to viewing the client against the plumb line, you should assess posture from the front and from the rear.

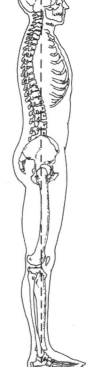

Figure 4.1 Line placement for the plumb line test.

Reprinted, by permission, from J. Griffin, 2006, *Client-centered exercise prescription*, 2nd ed. (Champaign, IL: Human Kinetics), 106.

Distinguishing Various Types of Faulty Postures

Identifying a client's postural deviations is important for two reasons. First, a client who exhibits one of the postural deviations (see the following list) would benefit from an evaluation by an orthopedic physician or a physical therapist. Some postural faults might warrant bracing or surgical interventions. Second, identifying the type of postural deviation will help pinpoint muscles that might require specific stretching or strengthening exercises. Deviations from the norm will indicate regions of the body that might be exposed to excessive forces. If this situation is not addressed with corrective exercises, these forces could contribute to the onset of injury.

Here are some common types of postural deviations (table 4.1):

■ *Scoliosis.* A scoliosis is a lateral and rotational curvature of the spine (figure 4.2). A scoliosis can be observed from behind, especially as the client bends forward. Recent evidence suggests that **idiopathic** scoliosis may be caused by genetic factors (Gao et al. 2007). Children and adolescents who present with a scoliosis should be referred to their physician for assessment. Adult clients with a scoliosis may be stable—that is, the degree of the curvature is not likely to increase. However, an adult client may also benefit from an orthopedist's or a physical therapist's evaluation. Clients are likely to have muscular tightness, especially in the region of the concavity. Stretching exercises may help the person maintain available flexibility and reduce muscle-related tension (although there is a lack of research evidence to support this claim).

■ *Kyphosis or a kyphotic spine.* Kyphosis is a curvature in the upper back that is frequently the result of postural adaptations. A kyphotic spine may also be the result of congenital factors or a thoracic vertebral fracture. This condition can also be a natural consequence of aging. When viewing the client from the side, as in the plumb line test, an individual who is kyphotic appears to have a large rounding of the upper back (figure 4.3).

■ *Sway back posture or excessive lordosis.* The normal convex orientation of the lumbar spine is inward, or toward the center of the body. When viewed from the side in the plumb line test, a person with a sway back posture usually presents with an exaggerated lumbar lordosis and, as a consequence, an excessive thoracic kyphosis. A client with a sway back posture might have tight low back muscles, tight hip flexors, and tight quadriceps. These clients often have significant abdominal weakness.

■ *Flat back.* Clients or patients who demonstrate a flat back posture will present with a loss (or decrease) of the normal kyphotic and lordotic curves (figure 4.4). When viewed from the side in the plumb line test, a person with a flat back posture will

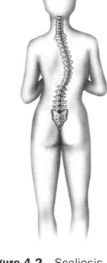

Figure 4.2 Scoliosis.

Reprinted, by permission, from W. Whiting and S. Rugg, 2005, *Dynatomy* (Champaign, IL: Human Kinetics), 65.

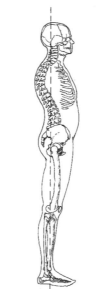

Figure 4.3 Kyphotic posture.

Reprinted, by permission, from J. Griffin, 2006, *Client-centered exercise prescription,* 2nd ed. (Champaign, IL: Human Kinetics), 106.

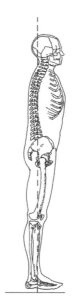

Figure 4.4 Flat back posture.

Reprinted, by permission, from J. Griffin, 2006, *Client-centered exercise prescription,* 2nd ed. (Champaign, IL: Human Kinetics), 106.

present with a loss of lumbar lordosis and possibly a loss of the normal curvature in the thoracic spine. A concern for clients with a flattened lumbar spine (or clients whose posture is progressing toward a *round back posture*) is the potential for excessive flexion moments on the lumbar discs. Repeated loading of the discs in this posture may increase the risk of disc injury in some people. Clients with a flat or round back are likely to have tightness of the hip flexors and hamstrings as well as generalized weakness of the core, especially the lumbar extensors.

Table 4.1 Postural Deviations and Associated Musculoskeletal Findings

Postural fault	Common musculoskeletal findings
Scoliosis	One or more lateral curves are present in the thoracic or lumbar spine. In the thoracic spine, a rib hump is present on the convex side. Muscular tightness is present on the concave side. Muscular weakness is possible throughout the core.
Kyphosis	Excessive kyphosis of the thoracic spine presents as a rounded upper or mid-back. Scapulae are likely to be protracted and possibly winging. The medial (middle) portion of the scapulae will appear as if they are lifted off of the back. Tight chest musculature (pectoralis major and pectoralis minor) and weak core and scapular musculature are often found in those with an excessively kyphotic spine.
Sway back	Excessive lumbar lordosis is present (and likely an associated level of excessive thoracic kyphosis). The client will likely have poor core strength. If excessive kyphosis is present, findings will be similar to those previously listed.
Flat back	The client displays a loss of normal thoracic kyphosis or normal lumbar lordosis. The client will likely present with core muscular weakness and a general loss of active range of motion of the spine.

Standing Active Range of Motion Testing

The following two tests are used to assess general mobility of the spine and hips. For the purposes of this testing, these movements are observed for quality of movement as opposed to being objectively measured.

Active Range of Motion Testing of the Spine

Objective: To assess the AROM of the lumbar spine

Client position: Standing

Provider position: Behind the client

Instructions: Tell the client to do the following:

1. Actively flex (bend forward).
2. Extend (bend backward).
3. Side bend (flex laterally).
4. Rotate.

Results: Observe for gross motion restrictions as well as side-to-side differences during side bending or rotation. A client may show a lack of flexibility by not having full range of motion or by demonstrating asymmetry of motion between sides.

Hip Crossover Test

The hip crossover test is an effective way to perform a quick assessment of a client's range of motion in the hips.

Instructions: Have the client stand on one leg. Tell the client to cross one leg (adduct and internally rotate the leg) in front of the other. Then have the client abduct and externally rotate the leg out to the side.

Results: Compare the movements on each side for symmetry.

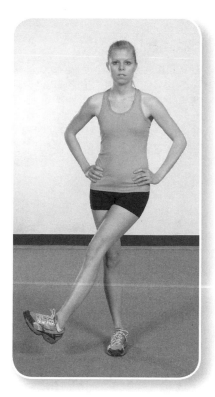
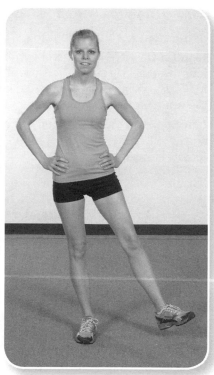

Standing Functional Testing

The functional tests performed in standing will allow you to assess the client's ability to perform functional movement patterns as well as to pinpoint potentially weak muscle groups. This information collected from these functional tests will help guide exercise prescription. The relative ease of performing these tests also allows you to quickly reassess the client in a few weeks in order to determine if the program you have initiated is helping to improve strength and function.

Squat Assessment

Instructions: Ask the client to perform a squat several times.

Results: From the front and from the side, observe how the client performs the squat. When viewing the client from the front, watch for symmetry of movement as the client lowers her body. When viewing the client from the side, observe the position of the spine in relation to the pelvis. Is the client able to maintain a neutral spine position? Does the client's hip move posteriorly when descending into the squat, or does the client instead use excessive knee flexion?

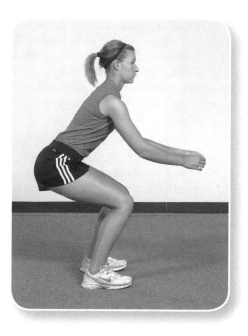

Lunge Assessment

Instructions: Ask the client to perform a forward lunge.

Results: Observe how the client performs the lunge. Core weakness may be present if the client bends the trunk to the side, adducts and internally rotates the hip, or shows valgus of the knee (the knee crosses the midline).

Variation: You may also want to conduct this test with the client lunging into other planes of motion that are deemed to be functionally important.

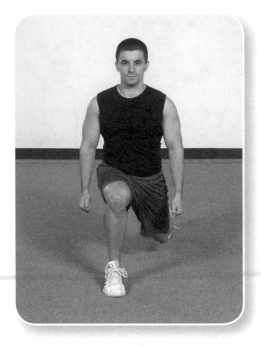

Single-Leg Squat Test

The single-leg squat test is a functional test that is useful for identifying dysfunctional hip strength and core control in clients and athletes (Zeller et al. 2003; DiMattia et al. 2005; Livengood et al. 2004).

Instructions: Ask the client to squat on one leg, having the client flex the knee to approximately 60°, then return to a full upright posture (Plastaras et al. 2005; Zeller et al. 2003). If the client is unable to maintain his balance during the test, that test is considered a failure and must be performed again.

Results: When observing the client from the front, you may be able to identify several dysfunctional movement patterns (see table 4.2). Ideally, when a client performs the single-leg squat, the pelvis will remain level. When an athlete has weakness in the hip abductors (e.g. gluteus medius), you are likely to see the opposite hip drop down. This is known as the Trendelenburg sign (DiMattia et al. 2005; Livengood et al. 2004).

For clients or athletes who demonstrate dysfunctional movement patterns in the single-leg squat, your intervention should be directed at strengthening the weak hip musculature (especially the hip abductors and external rotators). This should be followed by reintegrating the client into a functional strengthening routine.

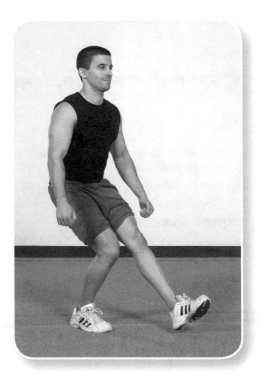

Table 4.2 Single-Leg Squat Malalignments and Related Dysfunction

Malalignment	Related dysfunction
Trendelenburg sign	Hip abductor weakness
Hip adduction or hip internal rotation	Weakness in the hip abductors and external rotators
Knee valgus	Hip weakness (or it may be inherent to the client's bony configuration)
Tibial internal rotation	Proximal hip weakness (or it may be inherent to the client's bony configuration)
Foot pronation	May be exaggerated by a proximally driven medial collapse (or it may be caused by the client's structural foot type)

Star Excursion Balance Test

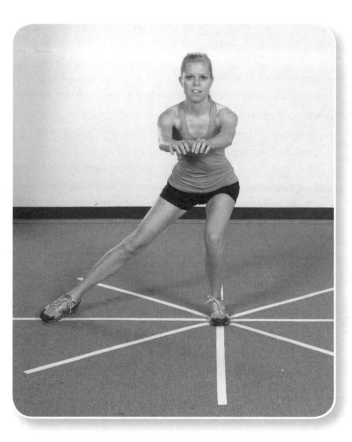

The star excursion balance test (SEBT) is a functional test designed to evaluate dynamic postural control. The SEBT is an easy test to perform and requires minimal setup time and materials. The star is created on the floor by placing four strips of tape on the floor—two in the shape of a plus sign (+) and two in the shape of a multiplication sign (i.e., a X). The strips forming the + and X should be positioned at 45° angles to each other (Gribble 2003). Each strip of tape should be approximately 8 feet long.

Instructions:

1. Have the client stand on one leg in the center of the star.

2. Instruct the client to reach as far as possible with the foot into each desired direction. The client should gently touch the ground with the forefoot without accepting weight onto the foot. The client should then return back to the starting point while maintaining the base of support with the stance leg.

3. Mark on the tape the point at which the client's foot makes contact. Measure this distance from the center of the star. If the client places weight on the foot, comes to rest, loses balance, or cannot return to the start position, the trial is discarded and should be repeated.

Results: Compare the symmetry of motion bilaterally. A lack of symmetry between sides may be associated with an increased risk for injury (Plisky et al 2006). The positions in which the client is not able to reach as far may suggest weakness in the gluteal muscles of the stance leg or dysfunctional dynamic balance.

TABLE OR MAT EVALUATIONS

After completing the standing assessment, ask the client to assume a supine position on a treatment table or elevated mat table. A series of tests will be conducted with the client in supine, prone, and side-lying positions.

Supine Positions

Testing the client in the supine position will provide valuable information regarding lower extremity flexibility. In addition, the flexor endurance test will be performed at this stage prior to progressing to the side-lying tests.

Hip Passive Range of Motion

Muscles tested: Hip internal and external rotators. In addition, this test position may provide information about the health of the hip (acetabulofemoral) joint. Clientele with significant asymmetry and pain on the side with significant range of motion loss should be referred to their medical provider for assessment. It is possible that the client has joint damage or arthritis.

Objective: To check for a lack of flexibility or an asymmetry of motion between hips

Client position: Supine with one leg positioned in the 90-90 position (hip and knee)

Provider position: Positioned to the side of the client. Place your hand (the hand that is closest to the client's head) on her thigh just above the knee joint. Place your other hand on the foot (near the heel) so that you can control the motion of the leg.

Instructions: Slowly rotate the foot either inward (medially) or outward (laterally) to assess the available internal and external range of motion of the hip. When you move the foot inward (or medially), you are actually testing external rotation at the hip. Likewise, when you move the foot outward, you are testing internal rotation at the hip.

Results: Assess for any lack of symmetry between sides. A decrease in motion suggests possible tightness of one or more pelvic or hip muscles. Further testing is necessary to identify specific muscles. If a loss of motion is present with a rehab patient, additional joint mobility testing for the hip and spine is warranted.

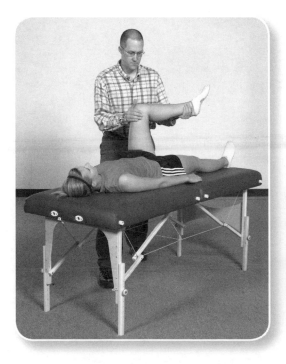
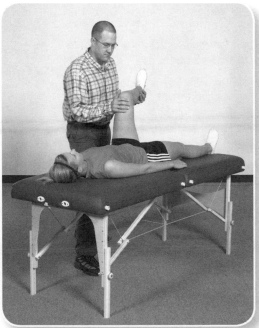

Straight Leg Raise Test

Muscles tested: Hamstrings

Client position: Supine

Provider position: Standing to the side of the table. Grasp the client's ankle with one hand while you palpate the front of the pelvis with your other hand.

Instructions: Slowly raise the client's straight leg to the point where you feel resistance or you feel movement at the pelvis.

Results: This test will allow you to assess a client's general hamstring flexibility and check for any lack of symmetry between sides. If the client complains of pain (not related to a general stretching sensation), the client should be referred to his medical provider.

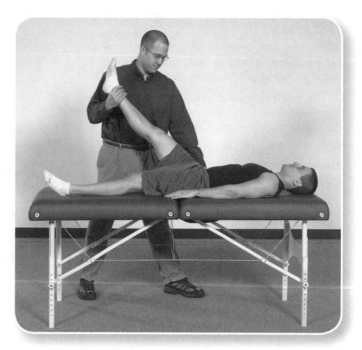

Thomas Test

Muscles tested: Psoas major, iliacus

Client position: Supine

Provider position: Kneeling (or standing) at the side of the table

Instructions: The client flexes and holds one hip while allowing the opposite thigh to rest on the table.

Results: If the hip presents with normal flexibility, the side tested will remain flat on the examining table. If the hip flexors are tight, the client's thigh will rise off the table.

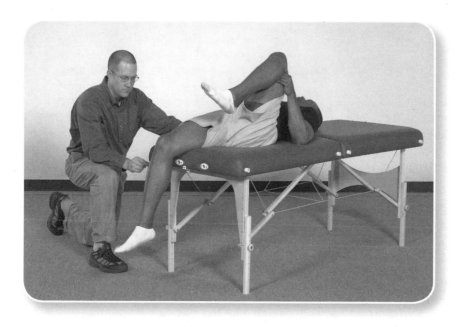

Flexor Endurance Test

Objective: To assess the functional endurance capacity of the anterior musculature of the core (rectus abdominis)

Client position: Reclined posture with her back initially resting against a bolster or a jig that is angled 60° from the table's surface (McGill 2002)

Provider position: Standing at the client's feet

Instructions:

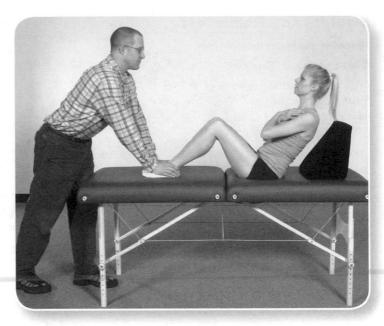

1. Ask the client to position herself with both hips and knees bent to 90° and the arms folded across the chest. A strap or belt may be placed across the ankles to help stabilize the body; however, instead of using the straps, you may provide support by manually stabilizing the client at the ankles.

2. To begin the test, remove the supporting object (bolster or jig), having an assistant slide the bolster 10 centimeters away from the client. Have the client hold this position as long as possible.

Results: Record how long (in seconds) the client is able to maintain this position. The test is stopped when any part of the client's back comes in contact with the bolster or jig. See table 4.3, page 49.

Side-Lying Positions

The following tests should be performed to each side of the body. The first test, the lateral musculature test, assesses endurance capacity for a few of the core muscles. The Ober's test will help identify a lack of flexibility on the lateral (outer) portion of the hip.

Lateral Musculature Test

Muscles tested: Obliques, transversus abdominis, quadratus lumborum

Client position: A side plank (or side bridge) pose with the top leg placed in front of the lower leg. The client will use the lower forearm and the feet to support herself.

Provider position: Standing in front of the client

Instructions: Keep track of how long the client can maintain the proper testing position.

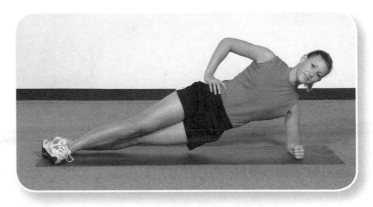

Results:

1. Watch first for an inability to assume a correct side plank position. This indicates a gross weakness of the lateral core muscles.

2. If the client is able to assume the correct position, record how long (in seconds) the client is able to maintain a straight posture. The client may attempt to adopt compensation strategies to maintain the position. Watch for the client's hips drifting toward the tabletop. Also observe whether the athlete cheats by rolling either forward or backward along the long axis of the body to maintain correct position. See table 4.3, page 49.

Ober's Test

Muscles tested: Tensor fasciae latae (TFL)

Client position: Side-lying position with the lower leg flexed at both the hip and the knee to provide stability

Provider position: Standing to the side of the table behind the client

Instructions: Passively raise the client's leg by abducting and extending the leg with the knee in a straight or flexed position (the knee may be flexed up to 90°). Next, slowly lower (or completely remove support for) the leg.

Results: If the TFL is tight, the leg will remain in an abducted position (instead of dropping toward the bottom leg).

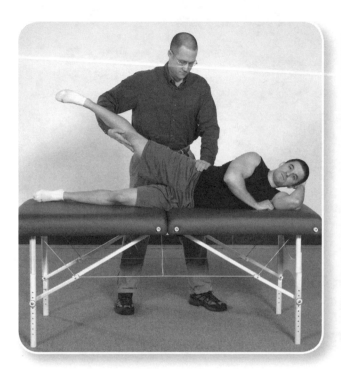
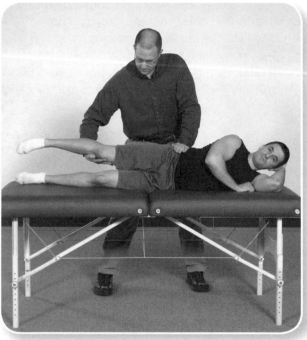

Prone Positions

The prone tests will provide information regarding hip flexibility and core endurance capacity of the extensor muscles.

Ely's Test

Muscles tested: Rectus femoris

Client position: Prone

Provider position: Standing to the side of the table

Instructions: Grab the client's ankle with your hand that is closest to his feet. Passively flex the client's knee, moving the ankle toward the buttock.

Results: If the hip flexes (or rises off the table) when you flex the knee, this indicates tightness of the rectus femoris muscle.

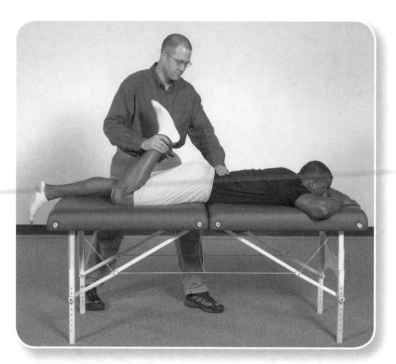

Back Extensor Test

Muscles tested: Erector spinae, multifidi

Client position: Prone with the torso positioned off the end of a treatment table (Biering-Sorensen 1984). Use a strap or belt to secure the client's legs to the table.

Provider position: Standing to the side in order to observe the client's torso alignment

Instructions: Tell the client to fold her arms across her chest so that her hands are resting on the opposite shoulders.

Results: Once the client is positioned correctly, record how long (in seconds) she is able to hold the position. The test ends once the client's body drops below the horizon. See table 4.3.

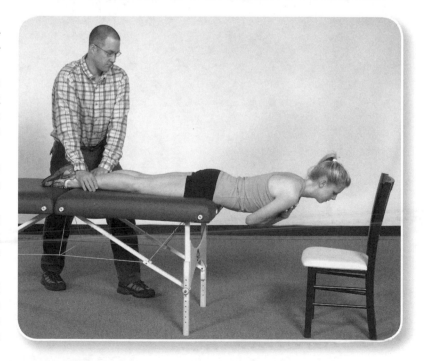

Variation: If a strap is not available, you (or an assistant) can use your body weight to stabilize the client's legs. Place a small chair or stool at the end of the table so that the client will be able to support and stabilize her upper body as she positions herself at the end of the table. Have the client lie prone on the table, and instruct her to scoot out to the end of the table. Place your arms or your body weight across her legs to stabilize the client. Begin timing once the client folds her arms across her chest. You should be able to observe when the client fatigues from this position. The chair is then available for the client to support herself again at the end of the test.

Helpful hint: Athletes and some other clients are very competitive and will attempt to maintain the testing position for as long as possible. Some clients may attempt to cheat by repeatedly performing back extension or hyperextension motions in order to maintain the position. If this occurs, stop the test even if the client's body has not broken the horizontal plane.

SCORING THE CORE ENDURANCE TESTS

Researchers have collected normative data for a few specific populations, but care should be taken to avoid comparing clients to this data. Table 4.3 presents average endurance times collected for healthy individuals with a mean age of 21 (McGill 2002). How then should scores be analyzed for a 16-year-old cross country athlete or a 45-year-old fitness client? Rather than expecting clients to have comparable endurance times, you should analyze the ratios between the time scores (table 4.4). When a muscular imbalance has been identified, exercise prescription should be directed toward improving the appropriate ratios.

Table 4.3 Mean Endurance Times for Healthy Individuals With a Mean Age of 21

Test	Males	Females
Extensor	161 seconds	185 seconds
Flexor	136 seconds	134 seconds
Lateral		
Right side	95 seconds	75 seconds
Left side	99 seconds	78 seconds

Data from McGill 2002.

Table 4.4 Ratio Scores Between the Endurance Tests

Endurance scores compared	Ratio suggesting imbalance
Right lateral endurance/left lateral endurance	> 0.05
Flexor/extensor endurance	> 1.0
Lateral endurance (either side)/extension endurance	> 0.75

Data from McGill 2002.

SUMMARY

The sequence of physical assessments presented in this chapter will help you recognize core dysfunction in your clients, athletes, or patients. Functional testing should begin with the client in a standing position, followed by supine, side-lying, then prone positions. Testing may reveal potential limitations in range of motion or flexibility and potential weaknesses in the torso or hip musculature. These findings must be interpreted to determine their functional significance. Integrating the assessment findings with the functional requirements for the client will help guide the core exercise program you develop for that client.

5

Fundamentals of Program Design

As a fitness or sports medicine professional, your goal is to implement optimal training strategies to help your clients achieve success. Exercise scientists have developed training protocols and strategies to maximize physical and physiological outcomes. Furthermore, exercise scientists are continually testing and refining these protocols. Your responsibility is to apply these evidence-based training methods and to incorporate your professional experience as you attempt to create a successful program for each client. This is easier said than done, especially when considering *core* program design. This chapter provides guidelines to help you improve your ability to design safe and effective core training programs.

NEEDS ANALYSIS

Before you begin training your client, you should complete a needs analysis. A 50-year-old client who had lumbar spine surgery 6 months ago is likely to have a different set of training goals than a 16-year-old athlete on the high school track and field team. These two individuals will require significantly different approaches to the design of a core exercise program. The results from the needs analysis will help guide your decisions when selecting exercises and implementing specific training variables. When performing a needs analysis, you should consider the client's training goals, current level of training, any history of musculoskeletal injury, and the results from the physical assessment and functional testing.

Client's Training Goals

By reviewing the client history form and interviewing the client, you should have a clear picture of the client's goals (see chapter 3 for a discussion of the initial client interview). During the needs analysis, you should restate these goals and have the client confirm them. Use these goals, along with the results of the physical assessment and functional testing, to guide your selection of core exercises and your development of a core training program.

For example, Jeremy, a 34-year-old accountant, wants to improve his overall fitness and join a city league basketball team next season. If his only goal were to improve his overall fitness, you'd probably select core exercises that have a difficulty level of basic to intermediate. But, since Jeremy wants to play in a basketball league, you may need to develop a program with intermediate to advanced core exercises as well as some low- to moderate-intensity plyometrics.

Client's Current Level of Training

Whether you are a personal trainer, a strength coach, or a rehabilitation specialist, many new clients who seek your services will probably not be currently participating in an adequate training program. If the client does participate in a regular exercise routine, you need to determine how many and what type of core stability exercises are included in that routine.

How intense should a client's exercise program be? Again, it depends on the client's goals. For most fitness and postrehab clients, a modest exercise routine with an emphasis on developing muscular endurance of the core will be appropriate (McGill 2002). Clients will tend to be more compliant with their exercise program if their routine is limited to three or four core exercises.

Overprescribing core exercises for these clients may limit the amount of time they have available for performing a comprehensive fitness routine. On the other hand, athletic individuals should be prescribed core exercises for strength and power in addition to core endurance exercises in order to meet functional demands.

History of Musculoskeletal Injury

As discussed in chapter 4, any client who is actively experiencing musculoskeletal symptoms should be referred to a medical provider for evaluation. However, you are more likely to be working with clients who have had an injury in the past but are not currently experiencing pain or other symptoms of injury. The client's history of injury can give you potential clues regarding underlying functional weaknesses. This will guide you in selecting appropriate core exercises. For example, a client may have experienced knee pain for several years. The pain may be partly attributed to functional weakness in the client's core, especially in the external rotators and abductors of the hip. Would it be appropriate to start this client's core program with plyometric exercises? Probably not. It would be better to concentrate on the client's functional weaknesses by prescribing exercises such as a side-lying leg raise, side bridge, and lunges. Another client may have had numerous episodes of back pain while trying to lift heavy objects. Is it appropriate to have this client begin with good mornings and bent-over rowing exercises? No. The client may have an underlying disc injury that is exacerbated by trunk flexion. Limited functional endurance in his back extensor muscles may also be contributing to his condition. So this client's program should initially focus on training core endurance in neutral spine postures, progressing toward functional goals as tolerated.

What is Plyometric Exercise?

Plyometric exercise is a style of exercise designed to improve power. Plyometric exercises consist of a quick stretch to the muscle or muscle group (eccentric action) followed by an immediate shortening contraction (concentric movement) of the same muscle or muscle group. The physiology behind plyometrics is explained in chapter 8.

Results From the Physical Assessment and Functional Testing

The results from your physical assessment and functional testing of the client will help guide your initial exercise prescription. For example, if the client demonstrates poor endurance capacity and muscular imbalances during the core endurance tests, training must be directed at correcting those deficiencies.

EXERCISE SELECTION

Using the information you have collected up to this point, you can now begin to design the client's program. Obviously, core stability training is only one component of the overall program you create.

Endurance Training for the Trunk

McGill has developed an evidence-based approach to developing a core training program for the trunk (2002). According to McGill's core exercise strategy, the first step must be to improve endurance capacity, especially any muscular imbalances. Reports have indicated that individuals with poor endurance capacity of the trunk as well as muscular imbalances (ratios between endurance scores) have an increased risk of back pain (McGill 2002; Biering-Sorensen 1984; Alaranta et al. 1995). A majority of clients with low back pain have poor core endurance capacity and muscular imbalances. In addition, many healthy and active clients frequently demonstrate poor core endurance. For example, many endurance athletes will describe a history of **intermittent** hip or knee pain. For these athletes, poor core stability may have contributed to a biomechanical situation that places the hips or knees at an increased risk of injury.

Muscular endurance is achieved by performing a high number of repetitions, usually with low loads. Figure 5.1 highlights the volume of repetitions necessary to achieve various training goals (Baechle et al. 2000). As you can see, to increase muscular endurance, a client needs to perform 12 or more repetitions per set.

To help clients improve the endurance of their torso muscles, you should have them perform a high volume of repetitions for each core exercise. A variety of endurance strategies are advocated

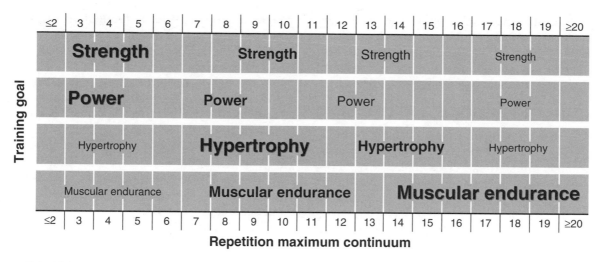

Figure 5.1 This continuum shows the number of repetitions needed to achieve various training goals. When performing fewer repetitions, a client can lift a heavier load.

Reprinted, by permission, from NSCA, 2008, Resistance training, written by T.R. Baechle, R.W. Earle, and D. Wathen, In *Essentials of strength training and conditioning,* 3rd ed., edited by T.R. Baechle and R.W. Earle (Champaign, IL: Human Kinetics), 401.

by sports medicine and strength training professionals. The program you ultimately design should be based on the needs of the particular individual you are training.

Training Tip

One effective endurance training strategy is to use the reverse pyramid training sequence (McGill 2004). For example, the side bridge exercise is routinely prescribed by strength training professionals in order to improve core endurance capacity in their clients. To use a reverse pyramid sequence in the side bridge exercise, the client would begin the sequence by performing five repetitions (holding each repetition for 10 seconds) of the side bridge exercise on one side, then immediately perform five repetitions on the opposite side. After performing five repetitions on each side of the body, the client would perform four repetitions (holding each for 10 seconds) of the exercise on each side of the body. During the final set the client would perform three repetitions of the same exercise on each side of the body.

Side Bridge Exercise: The client assumes a side-lying position with the forearm and elbow positioned under the shoulder. The client will then raise her body off the ground, supporting herself with only her forearm and feet. See page 64 for complete instructions for this exercise.

Strength Training for the Trunk

For postrehab clients or those who are only interested in improving their general health, a core endurance program for the trunk muscles will help them meet their goals. If a client has additional goals such as improving work or sport performance, strength training should also be incorporated into the program. To develop muscular strength, clients need to perform two to six sets of six or fewer repetitions (figure 5.1) (Baechle et al. 2000).

Flexibility Training for the Core

Maintaining or improving core flexibility is another important component of a core training program. Negative implications are associated with a general lack of functional flexibility. A lack of flexibility may impair a person's functional performance. For example, if a client is unable to effectively rotate through his core region, he may not be able to perform an optimal golf swing. Tight muscles can also interfere with optimal movement biomechanics, thus overstressing adjacent regions of the body and possibly contributing to injury.

To improve the flexibility of tight muscles, clients should perform stretching exercises on a regular basis. Static stretching exercises should be included at or near the end of the strength training program (see details in chapter 7). At that point, the muscles and connective tissues are warm. Clients should perform two or three repetitions of each stretch, holding each repetition for up to 30 seconds. In general, you should have your clients perform stretching exercises for less flexible regions of the body on a daily basis until the flexibility of that region has been optimized.

Plyometric Training for the Core

Most athletic individuals will benefit from the inclusion of plyometric exercises in their core training program. Plyometric exercises are key to developing the explosive power required to improve sport performance. Recent research has highlighted the functional benefits of including core plyometric exercises within an athlete's training program. For example, the inclusion of core-related plyometric exercises for golfers has contributed to improvements in club head speed during the swing and in driving distance of the ball upon impact (Doan et al. 2006; Fletcher and Hartwell 2004). Plyometric exercises have also been utilized to reduce the risk of traumatic knee injury in female athletes (Myer et al. 2006; Myer et al. 2008).

Numerous variables must be considered when implementing a plyometric training program. Chapter 9 provides details on each component of program design.

PRINCIPLES OF PERIODIZATION

Periodization is a strategy for program design that helps prepare and peak an athlete for competition (Wathen et al. 2000). This strategy involves deliberately manipulating the frequency, intensity, and duration of training in order to (1) prepare athletes for competition (preseason), (2) help them maintain their fitness during an extended season, and (3) allow them to taper their training during the off-season. A periodized strength training program is divided into cycles: macrocycles, mesocycles, and microcycles. A macrocycle spans the entire training period for the athlete. For most athletes, the macrocycle occurs over a 1-year period. But for some athletes, such as Olympians, macrocycles may extend over several years. A macrocycle is divided into several mesocycles. A mesocycle runs for a period ranging from several weeks to a couple of months. Finally, each mesocycle is divided into microcycles. The time period for a microcycle is 1 to 4 weeks. The exact number and length of the mesocycles and microcycles will depend on the training needs of the individual's sport. Periodization is a complex concept that requires concerted study and practice to master its application. The

recommended text for a detailed presentation of periodization is the National Strength and Conditioning Association's *Essentials of Strength Training and Conditioning, Third Edition* (2008, Human Kinetics). For the purposes of core training, the fitness professional needs to address how core stability exercises may be incorporated into each of the periodization phases.

A periodized training program may be classified by the sport season. These classifications include the off-season, preseason, in-season, and postseason. Within each season, specific training phases occur, requiring careful manipulation of the training variables.

The preparatory period (occurring during the off-season) is the time when an athlete has no scheduled competitions. The preparatory period is divided into three phases: the hypertrophy–endurance phase, the basic strength phase, and the strength–power phase (table 5.1) (Wathen et al. 2000).

The hypertrophy–endurance phase occurs during the first few weeks (1 to 6 weeks) of the preparatory period (Wathen et al. 2000). In this phase, the goal is for the athlete to develop muscular endurance capacity in preparation for the intense training that will come later. This is accomplished by performing high-volume, low-intensity training (figure 5.1). An appropriate strategy during this phase would be to build the athlete's trunk endurance capacity with exercises such as side bridges, crunches, and the bird dog (table 5.2). Instead of performing exercises that mimic functional movement patterns (e.g. squats (p. 83) and lunges (p. 68-71) during this stage, the athlete might perform a machine leg press or use other strengthening machines for the leg and hip to increase lower extremity strength. Near the end of this stage (weeks 5 and 6), the athlete could begin using low-intensity plyometrics for the core and lower extremities. The athlete should perform no more than 30 foot contacts (for a lower extremity jumping or hopping exercise) or 30 total throws (e.g. two-handed side throws to a rebounder, p. 125) per session during this phase of training.

The basic strength phase is designed to increase an athlete's muscular strength (Wathen et al. 2000). During this phase, the athlete may begin performing free weight exercises such as squats and lunges (exercises functionally similar to sports activities) using the intensity and volume variables presented in table 5.1. Tables 5.3a and 5.3b present a sample 3-day periodization model that highlights the training variables for this phase (for weeks 4 to 6, the

Table 5.1 A Periodization Model for Resistance Training

Period	Preparation → First transition			Competition			
	Hypertrophy and endurance	**Basic strength**	**Strength/power**	**Peaking**	**OR**	**Maintenance**	**Second transition (active rest)**
Intensity	Low to moderate	High	High	Very high		Moderate	Recreational activity (may not involve resistance training)
	50-75% 1RM	80-90% 1RM	87-95% 1RM 75-90% 1RM	≥93% 1RM		≈80-85% 1RM	
Volume	High to moderate	Moderate	Low	Very low		Moderate	
	3-6 sets	3-5 sets	3-5 sets	1-3 sets		≈2-3 sets	
	10-20 repetitions	4-8 repetitions	2-5 repetitions	1-3 repetitions		≈6-8 repetitions	

Reprinted, by permission, from NSCA, 2008, Resistance training, written by T.R. Baechle, R.W. Earle, and D. Wathen, In *Essentials of strength training and conditioning*, 3rd ed., edited by T.R. Baechle and R.W. Earle (Champaign, IL: Human Kinetics), 511.

Table 5.2 Sample Core Exercises Performed During the Hypertrophy–Endurance Phase

Exercise	Volume
Side plank (performed on each side)	3 sets each side × 10-second holds
Prone plank with hip extensions	3 sets × 10-20 repetitions performed bilaterally
Crunches	2-3 sets × 10-20 repetitions

Table 5.3a Sample Core Exercises Performed During the Basic Strength Phase: Weeks 1 to 3 (Monday, Wednesday, Friday)

Exercise	Volume
Lat pull-down	See table 5.1.
Squat	See table 5.1.
Lunge	See table 5.1.
Side plank (performed on each side)	3 sets each side × 30 repetitions
Prone plank with hip extensions	3 sets × 30 repetitions performed bilaterally
Crunches	30+

Refer to chapter 6 for descriptions of each exercise.

Table 5.3b Sample Core Exercises Performed During the Basic Strength Phase: Weeks 4 to 6 (Monday, Wednesday, Friday)

Exercise	Volume
Lunge (advance to multiple angles)	See table 5.1.
Cable chopping	30 repetitions each side
Cable one-arm rotation row	30 repetitions each side

Refer to chapter 6 for descriptions of each exercises.

athlete would continue the previous program and add the exercises listed in table 5.3b. Exercises such as squats, lunges, and lat pull-downs (p. 80, 83, and 81) would be subject to this model (table 5.3a and 5.3c). For this phase, you should choose core exercises from the intermediate and advanced categories (see chapter 6). For example, a program for a golfer could include the lunge twist (p. 83), the roman twist (p. 78), and the Russian twist (p. 79). The athlete may also advance to moderate-intensity plyometric exercises during this phase.

The strength–power phase is the final phase of the preparatory period. This phase often coincides with the athlete's preseason (up to the first event or game). The athlete's goals during this phase are to continue to increase strength and to develop power. Plyometric drills should be designed to replicate sport performance. Power exercises (full-body exercises that are performed quickly), such as the push press, would be added during this phase (Wathen et al. 2000). In this phase, the athlete should also continue to perform core exercises that replicate sport-specific movements.

In between each of the preparatory phases, the athlete should have a 1-week recovery period consisting of low-intensity, low-volume training (Wathen et al. 2000). During this time, the athlete should perform only two or three basic core exercises (2 or 3 sets with 10-second holds).

Table 5.3c Sample 3-Day Periodized Model for the Basic Strength Phase

Week	Sets	Rest period (min)	Reps	Monday 100% of assigned training load	Wednesday 80% of assigned training load	Friday 90% of assigned training load	Additional components of program T = Tuesday R = Thursday
1	3	3	8	80% 1RM	65% 1RM	75% 1RM	Endurance: T, R
2	3	3	6	80% 1RM	67% 1RM	77% 1RM	Endurance: T, R
3	4	3	6	85% 1RM	70% 1RM	80% 1RM	Endurance: T, R
4	4	3	6	85% 1RM	75% 1RM	83% 1RM	Endurance: T, R
5	5	3	5	90% 1RM and plyometric routine for lower body	70% 1RM	85% 1RM and plyometric routine for upper body	Endurance: T, R
6	5	3	5	90% 1RM and plyometric routine for lower body	75% 1RM	87% 1RM and plyometric routine for upper body	Running and core, 3 to 5 days a week

The competition period (in-season training) follows the preparatory period. During this period, the goal is for the athlete to peak—as well as preserve strength and power (table 5.1)—over the course of a few events or an entire season. Training volumes may be kept at a low to moderate level (2 or 3 sets of 6 to 8 repetitions), and training intensities should be no greater than the moderate level (80 to 85% of a 1-repetition max [1RM]) (Wathen et al. 2000). Others advocate a more intense competition period with training intensities greater than 90% of an athlete's 1RM; this would involve a low training volume (1 to 3 sets) for a small amount of repetitions (1 to 3). Power exercises, such as the push press and the clean and jerk, would be performed during this phase. Core exercises prescribed during this phase should include functional movement patterns (e.g. lunge with ball rotation, p. 85) and moderate- to high-intensity plyometrics (e.g. medicine ball sit-up, p. 129).

At the end of the athlete's competition period or sport season, the second transition period begins. This transition period runs up to the start of the next preparatory period. During this training period, the athlete is allowed to perform low-intensity, low-volume exercises (Wathen et al. 2000). The athlete should perform basic core endurance exercises during this period.

BALANCE TRAINING AND STABILITY TRAINING

Balance relates to a person maintaining her center of mass over her base of support. Balance training has applications ranging from rehabilitation (e.g.,

improving proprioception after an ankle sprain) to injury prevention (e.g., fall reduction programs). Balance training should not be confused with stability training. Stability training (or core stabilization training) uses exercises that enhance the function of the core to stabilize (or protect) the spine from potentially injurious forces. When prescribing certain balance training exercises, you may be able to incorporate core stabilization if an abdominal bracing technique is performed (McGill 2004).

SUMMARY

Once you have collected information from the interview, performed a needs analysis, and conducted the physical assessment, you are ready to design the client's individualized training program.

Muscular endurance training is often the primary goal for clients. For a majority of fitness and rehabilitation clients, a core training program that emphasizes muscular endurance will meet their functional needs. The core training program should address the muscles of the torso and the hips.

Strength training protocols should be added to core training programs for both traditional and industrial athletes. Core training programs for these individuals should initially include basic core endurance exercises to address any potential muscular imbalances, followed by the addition of moderate- to high-intensity core endurance and strengthening exercises. For competitive athletes, developing a periodized, year-round training program will help to maximize sports performance.

6

Core Exercises

Once you have completed the functional testing and have performed a needs analysis for your client, you are ready to begin selecting exercises for the client's training program. This chapter presents the core exercises that will improve your client's muscular endurance capacity and core strength. Later in this book, you will learn how to integrate the concepts of functional anatomy, client evaluation, and program design in order to enhance your ability to prescribe safe and effective core exercise programs. Chapter 9 will offer several sample training programs that illustrate core stability training in action.

ENHANCING CORE ENDURANCE AND STRENGTH

Core exercises improve the body's ability to minimize forces or loads applied to the spine. Most individuals—whether they are a patient, a healthy client, or an athlete—will benefit from the addition of core exercises to their overall training program. The exercises presented in this section will improve your clients' ability to stabilize their trunk.

The exercises in this chapter have been sorted into three categories based on their degree of difficulty: basic, intermediate, and advanced. The results obtained from the client's physical assessment will establish the starting point for an appropriate exercise prescription. A majority of rehabilitation patients and untrained clients should begin with basic core exercises. However, some of your clients may be able to safely perform a mix of basic and intermediate exercises. A core training program of intermediate exercises will meet the functional needs of most fitness clients and postrehab patients. Advanced core exercises are typically reserved for an athlete's training program.

Before a client performs any core exercises, you should provide him with basic information by discussing the functional anatomy of the core and the functional importance of core exercises. At this time you should also instruct the client on how to perform the abdominal brace. The abdominal brace is the cornerstone for all core exercises, so make sure your clients can correctly perform this crucial component. Educating your clients on the basics of core training may also improve their compliance with their exercise program.

The **abdominal brace** involves an isometric contraction of the musculature of the abdominal wall (with no inward or outward movement of the abdominal wall) along with a cocontraction of the lumbar musculature (McGill 2002). For each of the exercises discussed in this chapter, your client should initiate an abdominal brace before performing the movement. Two instructional techniques are recommended for teaching clients how to perform the abdominal brace (McGill 2002, 2004).

The first technique requires the client to actively participate while you provide instruction (McGill 2002, 2004). The client should assume a standing posture. Have the client slightly flex his lumbar spine (bend forward) while simultaneously palpating (touching) his lumbar extensors. Then instruct the client to extend himself upright while continuing to palpate his lower back muscles. Once the client obtains a posture in which his muscles feel like they are no longer contracting (or they feel relaxed), instruct the client to hold that position. Next instruct the client to perform the abdominal brace in this position. Once a client is able to perform the abdominal brace with this method, he should be able to perform the abdominal brace in any position. See the DVD for a demonstration of this technique.

Another way to teach a client the abdominal brace technique involves you and the client first performing a cocontraction of a peripheral joint (McGill 2002, 2004). For example, at the knee, you can demonstrate a cocontraction of the quadriceps and hamstrings. Asking the client to palpate (feel) your muscles both before and during your cocontraction will illustrate this technique. Next instruct the client to perform a similar cocontraction of the muscles of his knee joint. Repeat this technique as necessary until you determine that the client is able to demonstrate a cocontraction at any peripheral joint (the ankles, knees, elbows, and wrists are the most convenient joints to use for practice). Finally, ask the client to try to perform the cocontraction of the abdominal brace using the standing technique previously described.

Basic Core Endurance Exercises

Basic exercises can serve as a starting point for all core training routines. But don't let the "basic" classification fool you. These exercises will be challenging for many of your clients. For some, a routine of basic exercises will meet the needs for their particular fitness or postrehab goals. For others, once they have demonstrated the ability to successfully perform a basic core exercise routine, they should be advanced to an intermediate program.

Basic Quadruped Series

The core stabilization exercises performed in a **quadruped** position are excellent for training the spinal extensors and the gluteals.

Finding Neutral Spine in Quadruped

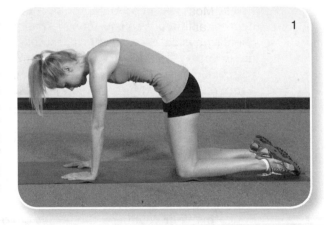

Starting position: Quadruped position (sometimes referred to as the table position)

Movement: The client first rounds her back toward the ceiling (the "angry cat" position or posterior pelvic tilt) then, reversing the position, she allows her pelvis to rotate toward the floor (the "camel" position or anterior pelvic tilt). The neutral spine position is considered the midpoint position between these two extremes of pelvic motion. Once the client has found her neutral spine posture, ask the client to perform the isometric abdominal brace.

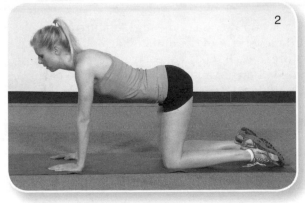

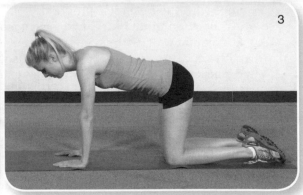

Common technique errors: In the quadruped position, many clients support their body weight primarily through their knees. To help clients improve their weight distribution, you should verbally and/or manually cue the client to share the weight equally among all four points of the "table." This equal weight distribution is vital to preventing compensation with the lumbar spine when the client attempts intermediate or advanced exercises.

Considerations for rehab clients: Clients must master this exercise before advancing to other basic and intermediate quadruped exercises. For some patients, their initial home exercise program may only consist of performing 10 repetitions of this exercise (holding each bracing contraction for up to 10 seconds) 3 times a day.

Considerations for fitness clients: These clients should quickly advance from this position to other basic or intermediate quadruped exercises that are more challenging.

Next exercise in progression: Quadruped position with arm raise or leg extension

Quadruped Position With Arm Raise

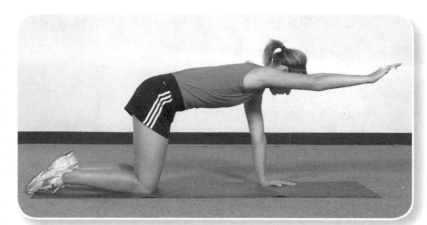

Starting position: Quadruped position

Movement: The client performs the abdominal brace and raises one arm in line with the torso. The client holds this position for a count of 5 to 10 seconds, returns to the starting position, and repeats the movement, alternating sides.

Considerations for rehab and fitness clients: This exercise is well suited for rehabilitation patients or deconditioned clients. Most will quickly master this exercise, and they can then be advanced according to their abilities.

Next exercise in progression: Quadruped position with leg extension or the bird dog exercise

Quadruped Position With Leg Extension

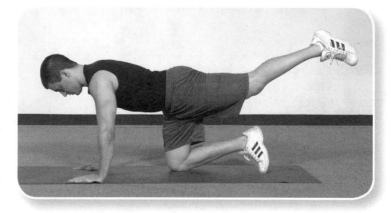

Prerequisites: For this exercise, the client must have significant strength in the gluteus maximus and must have the ability to stabilize the spine on the pelvis. The gluteus maximus is the main hip extensor used in this position. Gluteal strength is functionally important for both work-related tasks (lifting, squatting) and sport activities. If the client has difficulty performing the leg extension portion of this exercise, you may need to prescribe exercises that train the gluteus maximus in isolation (e.g., prone hip extension or bridging).

Starting position: Quadruped position with a neutral spine posture

Movement: The client performs the abdominal brace. Next, the client lifts the knee off the ground, contracting the gluteus maximus and extending the leg straight back. The goal is for the client to be able to extend the thigh (upper leg) in line with the trunk while maintaining a neutral spine.

Common errors:

1. The client does not fully extend the leg. To correct this error, instruct the client to extend (or raise) the leg back as far as he can while maintaining proper technique.

2. The client compensates by using other muscles to assist with extension. For example, an individual might compensate by side bending and rotating at the trunk in order to help achieve full leg extension. Correct this technique error by manually stabilizing the torso in the proper position as the client raises the leg.

Considerations for rehab and fitness clients: Cue the client, as necessary, to distribute his weight equally between each extremity before initiating the leg extension. If the client's weight is unevenly distributed to the legs, the client will shift his weight onto the supporting leg in order to raise the other leg.

Next exercise in progression: Quadruped opposite arm and leg raise (bird dog) (p. 65)

Basic Exercises to Strengthen the Glutes

Prone Hip Extension

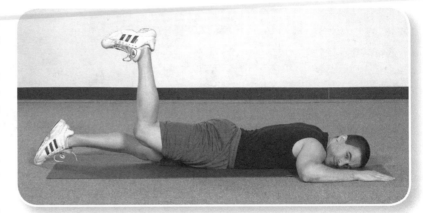

Starting position: Prone with both legs extended

Movement: The client bends (flexes) one knee to 90°. Next, the client contracts the gluteus maximus and lifts the foot toward the ceiling by extending the hip.

Common errors: The client compensates by extending through the lumbar spine.

Considerations for rehab clients: This exercise may cause pain in patients with facet joint irritation or degenerative joint disease in the lumbar spine.

Considerations for fitness clients: To strengthen the gluteus maximus, the client should perform 2 or 3 sets on each side for 15 to 20 repetitions.

Next exercise in progression: Bridging exercises, bird dog

Bridging

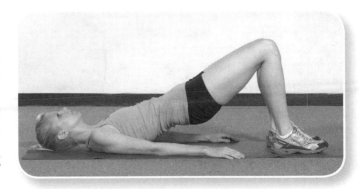

Starting position: Supine with the hips flexed to 45° and the knees flexed to 90° (hook-lying position). The feet should be flat on the ground and shoulder-width apart.

Movement: The client contracts the glutes and lifts (bridges) the hips toward the ceiling. The hips should rise to the point where the thighs, hips, and back are all in a straight line (avoiding hyperextension in the lumbar spine).

Common errors:

1. The client arches the back by hyperextending the lumbar spine. This often results from a lack of proprioceptive control. Attempt to correct this technique error by verbally cueing the client. If the client continues to hyperextend through the lumbar spine, she might require additional training with the prone hip extension and the quadruped position with leg extension exercises.

2. Some clients may initiate the bridging motion by contracting their hamstrings. The

hamstrings, known for their primary role as knee flexors, also assist with hip extension. When the hips are weak or dysfunctional, clients will compensate by contracting the hamstrings first. To help correct this error, as the client performs the bridge, you can palpate the hamstrings while cueing the client to contract the glutes. The client may benefit from additional hip extension strengthening with the prone hip extension exercise and the quadruped position with leg extension exercises.

Next exercise in progression: Intermediate bridging exercises (p. 66)

Clamshell

The clamshell exercise facilitates activation of the gluteus medius (McGill 2004).

Starting position: Side-lying position with the hips slightly flexed and the knees bent to approximately 90°

Movement: The client raises the top knee off of the bottom knee by contracting the hip muscles. This exercise mimics the opening of a clamshell. The movement should be isolated to external rotation of the hip.

Common errors: To raise the top knee, clients will sometimes compensate by rolling at their trunk or rotating their pelvis. Cue these clients to avoid rolling or rotating at their torso or pelvis as they lift their knee. You can also stabilize their pelvis and low back with your hands. This may help clients isolate movement to lateral hip rotation.

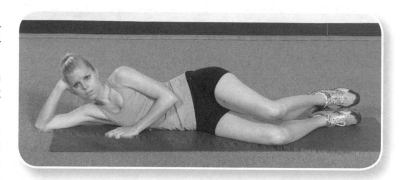

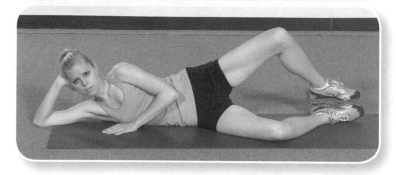

Considerations for rehab and fitness clients: Once a client is able to correctly perform the clamshell exercise with hip external rotation, the client should advance to the next series of exercises.

Next exercise in progression: Side-lying straight leg raise

Side-Lying Straight Leg Raise

Starting position: Side-lying position with both legs extended

Movement: The client abducts (raises) the top leg. This leg should be externally rotated slightly (10 to 20°). The client should elevate the leg as high as possible; the movement occurs at the hip joint, and the torso is kept in a neutral position.

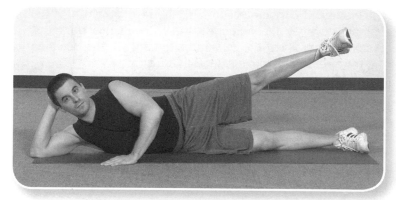

Common errors:

1. The client activates the hip flexors in order to compensate for weak hip abductors.
2. The client abducts the leg while the foot (or leg) is internally rotated.

To help correct these errors, have the client assume the starting position with a heel placed against the wall. The client should abduct the leg while keeping the foot against the wall throughout the exercise movement. This technique helps the client develop the appropriate strategy for motor control.

Basic Exercises in a Standing Position

Straight-Arm Pull-Downs

Starting position: Standing while facing a cable machine. Both shoulders are forward flexed to 90°, and the client is holding on to a lat bar with an overhand grip. The scapulae (shoulder blades) should be retracted and depressed.

Movement: The client pulls the lat bar toward the legs, holds the position for 1 or 2 seconds, then slowly returns the bar to the starting position.

Common errors: Rehab or fitness clients may be unable to maintain a neutral spine posture throughout the motion. To correct this error, reduce the weight to one that allows the client to perform the exercise while maintaining a neutral spine.

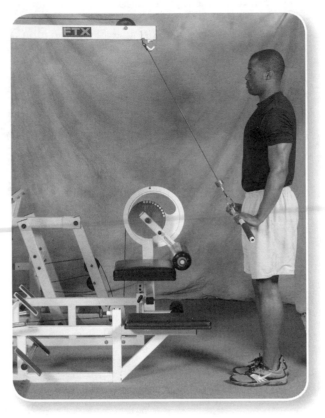

Wall Lean

The wall lean (also known as the side bridge remedial exercise) is a preparatory exercise for the side bridge progression. *Not all of your clients will need to perform this exercise.* This exercise is ideal for senior clients (who may have difficulty rising from the floor) or individuals who are rehabilitating from a low back injury or from spine surgery. For some clients, such as geriatric clients or those who are severely deconditioned, the wall lean may be the primary exercise for training the quadratus lumborum, the obliques, and the transversus abdominis (McGill 2002).

Starting position: Standing with the arm at shoulder level and the forearm placed on a wall. The client leans against the wall, supporting the body with the forearm.

Movement: The client holds this position for up to 10 seconds (2 or 3 sets on each side).

Next exercise in progression: Cable side steps or the side bridge (p. 64)

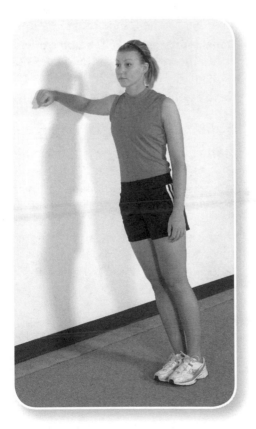

Cable Side Steps

If a client finds the wall lean too easy but is unable to assume a side-lying position on the floor, cable side steps are a good option.

Starting position: Standing while holding the cable or exercise band in front of the abdomen

Movement: The client takes five side steps away from the machine and holds this position for 5 to 10 seconds. The client then takes five side steps back to the starting position.

Variation: If a cable machine is not available or feasible, a resistance band can be used for an adequate level of resistance.

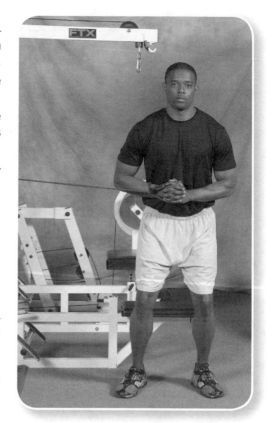

Additional Basic Exercises

Crunch

The crunch and its many variations can be used to train the abdominal muscles, specifically the rectus abdominis. When first learning the crunch, the client must be supervised closely. Clients often make numerous errors in technique when performing the crunch.

Starting position: Supine with the legs in a hook-lying position

Movement: The client performs the crunch by contracting the rectus abdominis while bending (crunching) through the mid-back region. The client's arms may be placed alongside the torso, across the chest, or alongside the head.

Common errors:

1. The client places the hands behind the head. Although some clients may be able to place both hands behind the head to support it, others may inadvertently apply a potentially harmful force to the head (McGill 2002). Thus, you should avoid instructing clients to place their hands behind their head.

2. The client does not keep the head and neck in alignment with the upper torso.

3. The client rises too far into the crunch. A client with a weak rectus abdominis may try to use the hip flexors, performing a sit-up instead of a crunch. You should cue the client to avoid "overcrunching" by limiting his rise to only the shoulder blades.

Key tip: The crunch exercise is preferable to the sit-up exercise. The sit-up increases lumbar flexion, which may provoke symptoms in an individual who has a history of disc injury.

Next exercise in progression: Intermediate exercises for the rectus abdominis (p. 67, 71)

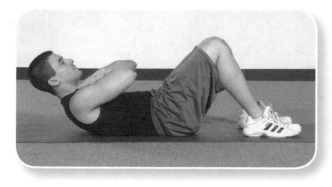
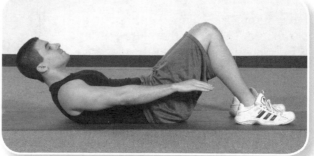

Side Bridge (Beginner)

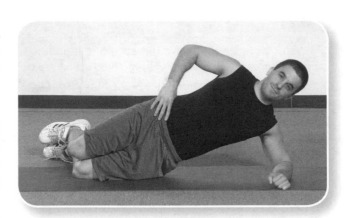

Starting position: For the basic (or beginner) version of this exercise, the client lies on his side with his body in the presupport position (on the forearm, hip, and thigh), with the knees bent.

Movement: The client performs an abdominal brace, raising his hip and thigh off the table or floor. In the terminal position, the forearm, knee, and leg should support the body weight. The client should hold this posture for up to 10 seconds on each side for the desired number of repetitions.

Considerations for rehab and fitness clients: The basic (beginner) version of the side bridge is a valuable training option for rehabilitation clients as well as for clients who are generally deconditioned. This exercise is ideal for facilitating strengthening of the obliques, the transversus abdominis, and the quadratus lumborum.

Next exercise in progression: To progress from this beginner position toward the intermediate exercise, the client should gradually extend his legs (p. 66).

Front Plank or Prone Plank (Basic Position With or Without Knee Supports)

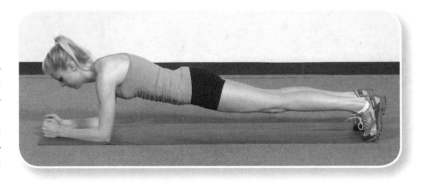

Starting position: Prone position with the body being supported by the forearms and the toes. The torso, hips, and legs should be in alignment. If a client has difficulty assuming this position, she may support her body with her knees.

Movement: The client holds this pose for 10 seconds and then rests. The client repeats the movement for the desired number of repetitions.

Next exercise in progression: Front plank with arm or leg extension (p. 67)

Straight Leg Raise

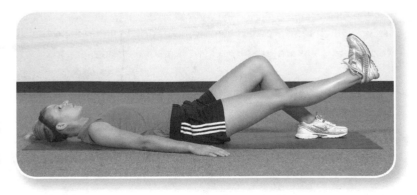

Starting position: Supine position with one leg resting on the floor with the knee in full extension. The other hip is flexed to approximately 60 degrees.

Movement: The client contracts the muscles of the thigh then lifts the leg 6 to 8 inches off the floor holding this position for up to 5 seconds. The client repeats the movement for the desired number of repetitions. This exercise strengthens the anterior muscles of the hip.

Intermediate Core Endurance Exercises

Quadruped Opposite Arm and Leg Raise (Bird Dog)

The quadruped opposite arm and leg raise—also known as the bird dog (McGill 2002)—is an exercise that is frequently prescribed by strength coaches and rehabilitation specialists. For this intermediate exercise, the client must have the ability to coordinate the elevation of the opposite arm and leg while maintaining a neutral spine.

Starting position: Quadruped position with a neutral spine. The client should be performing an abdominal brace.

Movement: The client raises one arm and simultaneously raises the opposite leg. The client holds the position for 5 to 10 seconds. Repetitions should be performed to each side.

Common errors:

Novice clients will rarely be able to perform this exercise correctly. For your clients to be successful with this exercise, you may need to supplement their training program with several basic core exercises in order to isolate weak musculature (table 6.1).

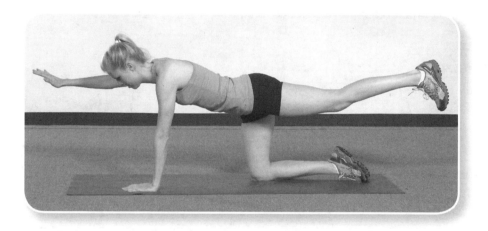

Table 6.1 Muscle Weakness Patterns Affecting the Bird Dog Exercise

Muscle or muscle group	Dysfunctional movement pattern	Corrective exercise
Erector spinae	Unable to lock the spine on the pelvis (Observe the client side bending, rotating, or arching the trunk.)	Straight-arm pull-downs, front planks
Gluteus maximus	Unable to fully extend the hip	Prone hip extension, bridging
Gluteus medius and minimus	Unable to fully extend the hip	Clamshell, side-lying straight leg raise
Rectus abdominis	Unable to lock the spine on the pelvis	Front planks, crunches

Side Bridge (or Side Plank) Exercise

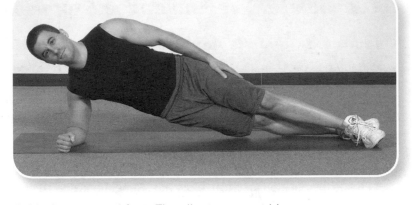

The side bridge (also known as the side plank) is the next progression after the client has mastered the basic (or beginner) side bridge pose.

Starting position: Side-lying position with the forearm and elbow positioned under the shoulder. The feet may be positioned one in front of the other or with one on top of the other.

Movement: The client raises his body off the ground, supporting himself with only his forearm and feet. The client may rest his top arm on his torso.

Common errors: The client's movement includes subtle torso rotations, or the client is unable to maintain the hips in a neutral position. Observe the client to ensure that the head, torso, and legs are in alignment.

Next exercise in progression: Side bridge with hip abduction (p. 76)

Bridging With a March

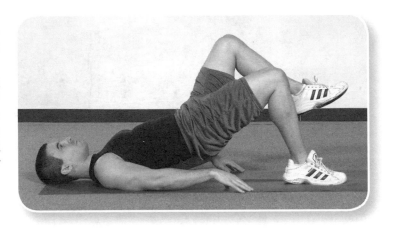

Starting position: Supine with the legs in a hook-lying position

Movement: The client performs a bridge. At the top of the bridge, the client "marches" by slightly flexing one hip, holds the position for 5 to 10 seconds, then lowers the leg to return to the starting position. The client should alternate sides for the desired number of repetitions.

Bridging With Leg Extension

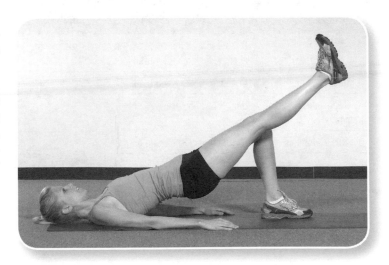

Starting position: Supine with the legs in a hook-lying position

Movement: The client first performs a bridge. At the top of the bridge, the client straightens (extends) one knee, maintaining a straight line from the shoulder through to the ankle. The client holds the position for 5 to 10 seconds. The client should alternate sides for the desired number of repetitions.

Front Plank

Starting position: Supporting the body with the forearms and feet while maintaining the core in a neutral alignment

Movement: The client holds this position for 10 seconds. The client should repeat this for the desired number of repetitions.

Key tips: Monitor the client's alignment during the movement portion of the exercise.

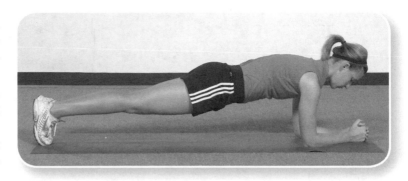

Common errors: The client is unable to maintain proper alignment—the client either flexes at the hips or sticks the buttocks up toward the ceiling.

Next exercise in progression: Front plank with arm or leg extension

Front Plank With Arm or Leg Extension

Starting position: Same as the front plank

Movement: From the front plank position, the client lifts one arm or one leg. The client holds this position for 5 to 10 seconds and then repeats to the opposite side.

Considerations for fitness clients: This is an excellent exercise for endurance athletes. Performing the front plank with leg extension for multiple sets and high repetitions will improve core endurance as well as strengthen the hip extensors.

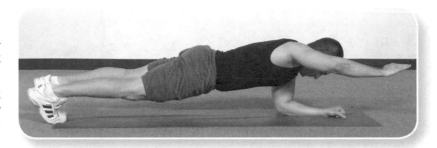

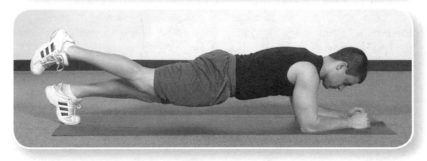

Front Plank With Opposite Arm and Leg Extension

Starting position: Same as the front plank

Movement: The client simultaneously elevates one arm and the opposite leg, holding this position for 5 to 10 seconds. The client should perform multiple repetitions on each side.

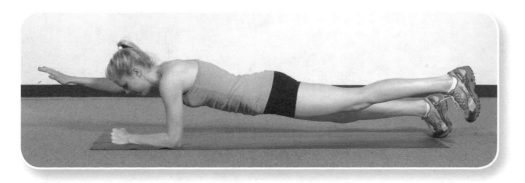

Role of Medicine Balls and Physioballs in Core Endurance Training

The medicine ball and physioball can be incorporated into a dynamic core stability program using partner drills and plyometric exercises (see chapter 8). The advantage of using medicine balls or physioballs is that they enable a person to train the core muscles in specific movement patterns that can't be performed with traditional free weights and machines. However, this equipment should be used judiciously. The client's goals and assessment results should be used to determine whether medicine balls or physioballs are appropriate for the client's program. Does a 55-year-old sedentary client really need to perform plyometric medicine ball throws? What is the functional benefit of the over-under drill for a 35-year-old sedentary accountant?

Obviously, a disadvantage is that the client must have access to a physioball, a medicine ball, a plyometric rebounder, and a partner! Because many of the following exercises require the use of equipment or a partner, these exercises should be used primarily to supplement a client's core exercise program.

Standing Torso Rotation

Starting position: The client and the partner stand facing opposite directions with their bodies separated by the distance of each other's arms.

Movement: The client initiates the movement by rotating toward the right side while holding the medicine ball at waist level. The partner receives the ball by rotating toward his left side. The exercise continues as the partner changes direction, rotating toward the right side. This sequence is repeated to each side for the desired number of repetitions.

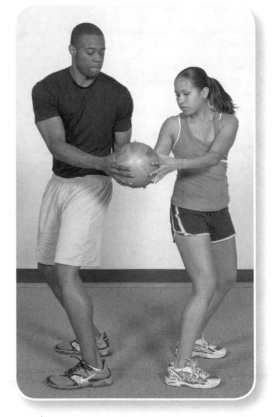

Standing High-Low Torso Rotations

Starting position: The client and the partner stand facing opposite directions approximately 1 to 2 feet (30 to 60 cm) away from each other. The client holds the medicine ball near her right hip.

Movement: The client starts by rotating the ball from her right hip diagonally across her body toward her left shoulder. The partner rotates toward her right side to receive the medicine ball from the client. The partner then moves the ball from the "high" position, lowering the ball across her body to the opposite side. The client mirrors this movement, receiving the ball in the "low" position.

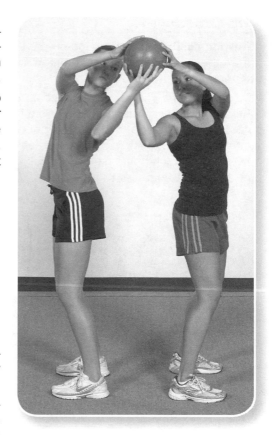

Over-Unders

Starting position: The client and the partner stand approximately 1 to 2 feet apart from each other, facing opposite directions.

Movement: The client raises the medicine ball overhead, handing it to the partner. The partner grabs the ball and lowers it to between his legs in order to hand it to the client. The pair should perform a set number of repetitions in one direction; they should then repeat the drill, reversing directions.

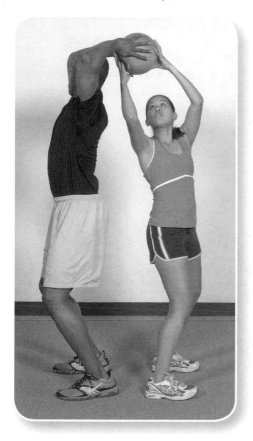

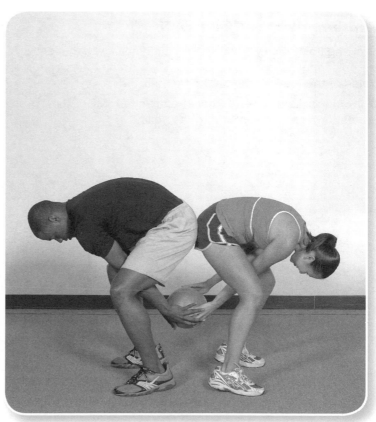

Hip Crossover

Starting position: Lying supine on the ground with outstretched arms and with the legs (from the knees to the feet) resting on a physioball. The hips and knees are both flexed to approximately 90°.

Movement: The client rotates the ball to one side while keeping the ball on the ground throughout the exercise. The client should only rotate as far as she can while still keeping her upper back and shoulders flat against the surface. The goal is for the client to touch the ground—or come as close as possible—with her *ipsilateral* knee (the knee on the side to which she is rotating). The client should perform this exercise to each side for the desired number of repetitions.

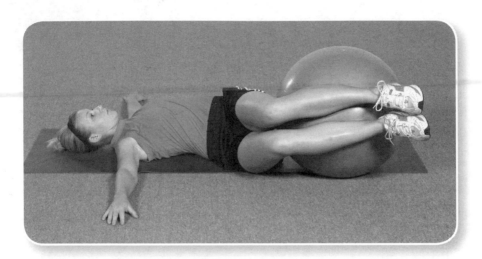

Bridging With a Physioball

Starting position: Lying supine on the ground with the feet on a physioball. The feet may be positioned in one of two ways: (1) with the heels contacting the ball or (2) with the soles of the feet resting flat on the ball.

Movement: As in the traditional bridging exercise, the client squeezes (contracts) the glutes to raise the hips toward the ceiling.

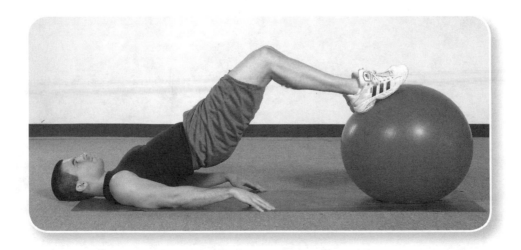

Reverse Crunch

Starting position: Lying supine on the ground with both legs straight. The client's ankles will straddle a physioball.

Movement: The client brings the knees toward the chest, lifting the ball off the floor.

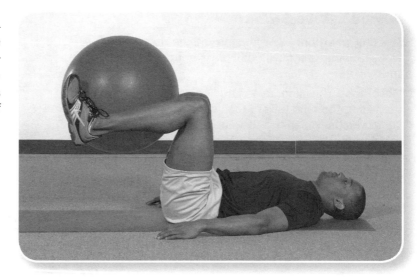

Knee Tuck on a Physioball

Starting position: A push-up position with the palms on the floor to support the upper body. The shins are resting on top of the physioball.

Movement: The client pulls the knees toward the chest, allowing the physioball to roll forward. The client's toes will be on top of the physioball at the end of the tuck. The client holds this position for 5 seconds. The client then returns to the starting position by extending the legs, rolling the ball away from the body.

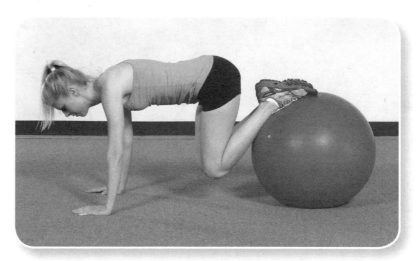

Crunch on the Physioball

Starting position: Lying on the back with the feet resting on top of a physioball. The hips are in line with the torso and the knees are flexed to 90°.

Movement: The client performs a crunch in a similar manner to a traditional crunch.

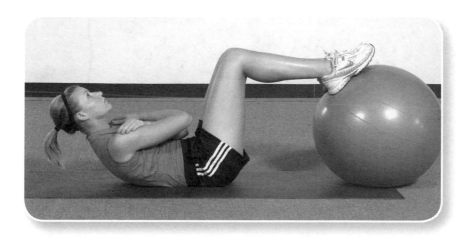

Physioball Leg Raise

Starting position: Lying supine on the floor and grasping the physioball with both feet and ankles

Movement: The client raises the legs straight up, flexing the hips toward 90° while keeping the lower back against the floor. The client holds the position for 5 to 10 seconds, then lowers the ball to the floor.

Key tips: Many clients will be unable to flex the hips to 90°. Allow these clients to flex the hip as high as possible while keeping the low back flat on the floor.

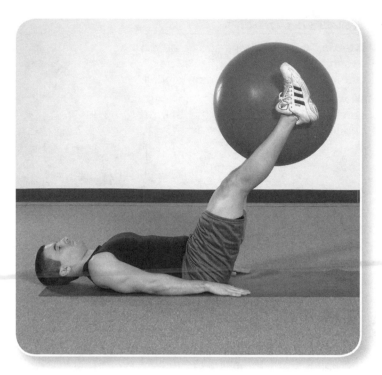

Ball Plank Twists

Starting position: A plank-like position with the palms flat on the floor (directly under each shoulder) to support the upper body. The feet should be resting on top of the physioball.

Movement: The client rotates to one side, moving the left hip up toward the ceiling, and holds this position for 2 to 3 seconds. The client then returns to the starting position and reverses directions. The client should perform the desired number of repetitions to each side.

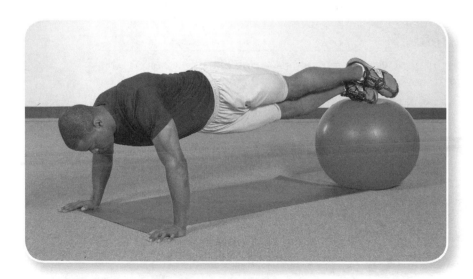

Bench Press on a Physioball

Starting position: Lying supine on top of the ball with the hips and thighs in line with the torso, the knees flexed to 90°, and the feet flat on the ground. A spotter stands nearby to hand the client a dumbbell for each hand.

Movement: The spotter hands the weights to the client's outstretched arms. The client slowly lowers the arms, allowing the elbows to flex to 90°. The client repeats the sequence, performing the bench press with dumbbells while maintaining a neutral spine position.

Common error: If the client is frequently unable to maintain a neutral spine, this may indicate that the client is attempting to press too much weight.

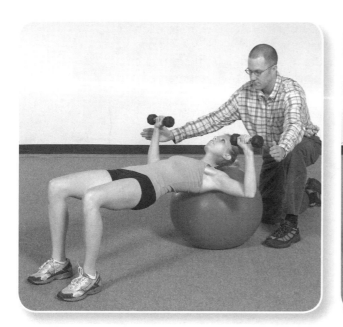
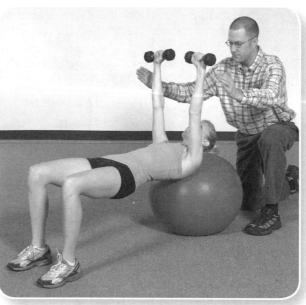

Shoulder Press on a Physioball

Starting position: Seated on the physioball with the hips and knees flexed to approximately 90°. A spotter should assist the individual with this exercise, especially when heavy weights are lifted.

Movement: The client performs a shoulder press while maintaining a neutral spine posture.

Common error: If the client is unable to maintain a neutral spine posture during the lift, this may indicate that the client is attempting to press too much weight.

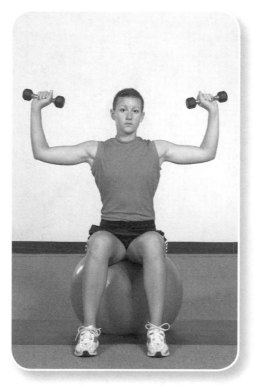
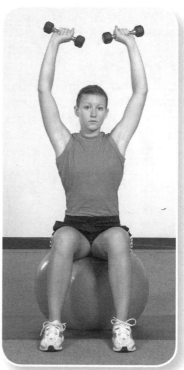

Advanced Core Endurance Exercises

The exercises in this section are generally prescribed to athletes, performing artists, and high-level clients.

Side-Lying Bilateral Leg Raise

Starting position: Side-lying position with both legs extended

Movement: The client raises both legs 2 to 4 inches (5 to 10 cm) off the ground, holding this position for 5 to 10 seconds. The client then lowers the legs to the starting position and repeats the movement for the desired number of repetitions.

Next exercise in progression: If a client is able to perform this exercise with excellent technique, progress him to the double-side jackknife. To perform the double-side jackknife, the client raises both the legs and the trunk (elevating the upper portion of the torso) at the same time. The client holds the position for 5 to 10 seconds and then returns to the starting position. Repeat for the desired number of repetitions on each side.

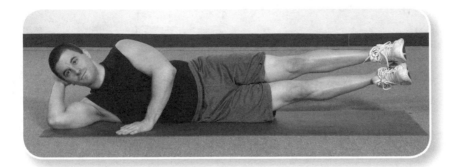

Jackknife on a Physioball

Starting position: Plank position with the hands or forearms in a neutral position on the floor, supporting the upper trunk. The legs are supported at the shins by a physioball.

Movement: The client uses the legs to draw the ball toward the body while raising the hips toward the ceiling. The client holds the position for 5 to 10 seconds and then returns to the starting position.

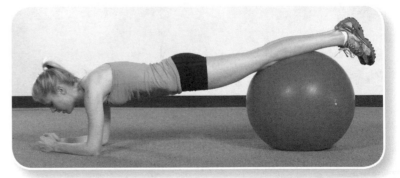

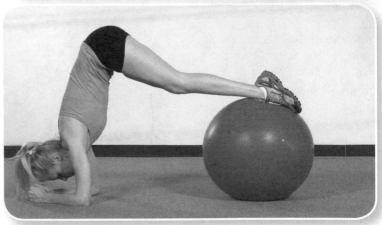

Inverted Hamstring

The inverted hamstring exercise addresses hamstring tightness, improves core stabilization, and incorporates balance training.

Starting position: Balancing on one leg, with the knee in full extension, while maintaining optimal posture

Movement: The client bends at the hips (not the waist) while maintaining a straight (neutral) spine. The client's arms should be outstretched to the sides to assist with balance. As the client leans forward, she will feel a stretching sensation in the hamstrings.

Common error: Clients with significant hamstring tightness will have the tendency to compensate by either rounding or rotating at the lower back.

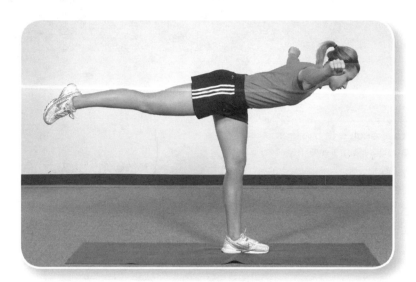

Hang Twist

Starting position: Gripping a pull-up bar or the top of a squat rack with both hands using an underhand grip

Movement: The client raises the knees toward the right shoulder until the thighs are parallel with the floor. The client holds the position for 1 or 2 seconds, then lowers the legs under control. The client then repeats the movement to the opposite side.

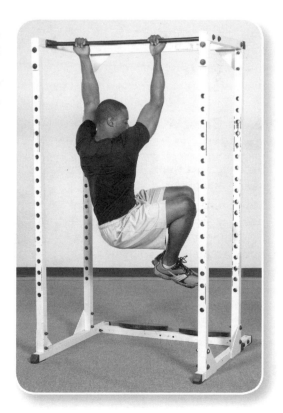

Prone Twist

Starting position: Both feet are placed on a bench with both hands placed on the floor, shoulder-width apart

Movement: The client bends one knee to waist height and then rotates the trunk toward the opposite side, holding this position for up to 5 seconds. The client then switches legs and repeats the movement to the opposite side.

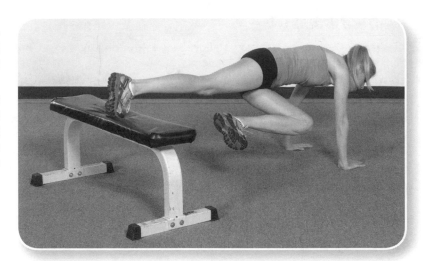

V-Ups

Starting position: Lying flat on the back with the legs extended and the arms positioned straight overhead

Movement: The client simultaneously raises the torso and the legs, creating a V shape. The hands should reach toward the feet at the top of the movement. The client should then return to the starting position, slowly lowering the body into a supine position.

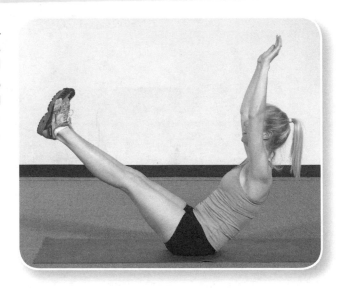

Side Bridge With Hip Abduction

Starting position: Same as the side plank (intermediate)

Movement: While in the side plank position, the client abducts the top leg, lifting it off of the bottom leg approximately 6 to 8 inches. The client holds this position for up to 5 seconds.

Variation: Hip flexion can be used instead of abduction. Once the client has assumed the side plank position, instruct him to flex at the

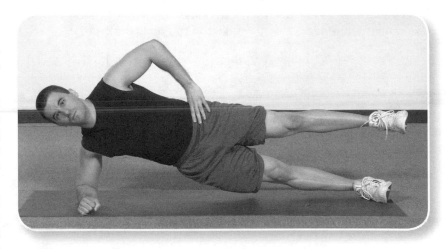

hip, bringing the knee toward the chest. When the client's hip and knee are both in a 90-90 position, he holds the position for up to 5 seconds.

Side Bridge With Shoulder External Rotation

Starting position: Same as the side plank (intermediate). A towel is placed between the client's elbow and torso. Placing the towel here will help to position the shoulder in an optimal training position and cue the client to keep his elbow by his side.

Movement: While in the side plank position, the client holds a light dumbbell with the shoulder and elbow in a 90-90 position. Instruct the client to externally rotate the shoulder.

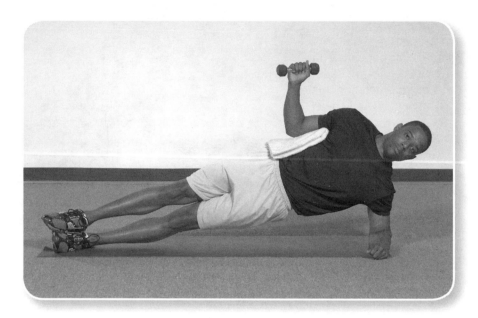

Three-Point Plank With Upper Extremity Exercise

Starting position: A three-point plank posture in which the client is supporting the body with both feet and one extended arm.

Movement: While in the three-point plank position, the client performs an upper extremity exercise with the free arm. This exercise may be a shoulder flexion, shoulder horizontal abduction, shoulder row, or shoulder extension exercise.

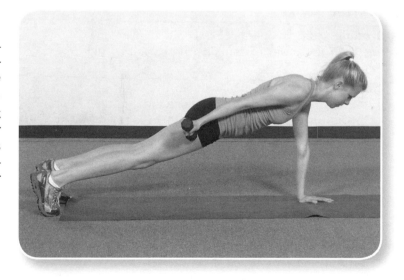

Roman Chair

Starting position: Secured in a roman chair. The client's feet should be under the supports, and the chair should be adjusted to allow the client to bend completely forward at the waist.

Movement: The client raises the torso from a flexed position to a neutral position.

Considerations for rehab clients: Hyperextending the spine at the top of the movement is usually not necessary and is contraindicated for patients with spondylolisthesis or degenerative joint disease. You must also weigh the risks of incorporating this exercise for an individual with a history of disc-related pain.

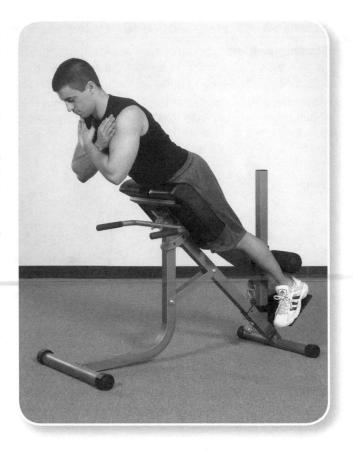

Roman Twist

Starting position: Maintaining a neutral spine posture with the lower extremities supported by the roman chair

Movement: In an upright position, the client performs a twist (trunk rotation) to one side, returns to the starting position, then performs the twist to the opposite side.

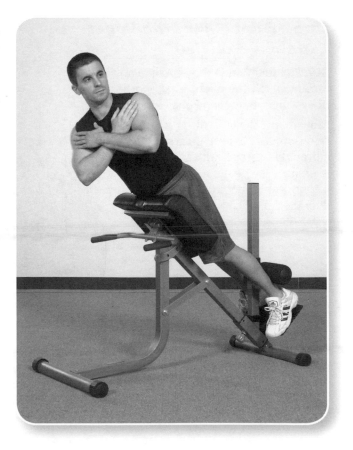

Russian Twist

Starting position: Positioned on the roman chair as shown

Movement: The client maintains the abdominal bracing contraction while slowly rotating the trunk and arms to the side. After rotating to the side, the client holds the position for up to 5 seconds. The client then returns to the starting position and repeats the movement to the opposite side.

Variation: To increase the challenge of the exercise, the client can hold a medicine ball out with straight arms.

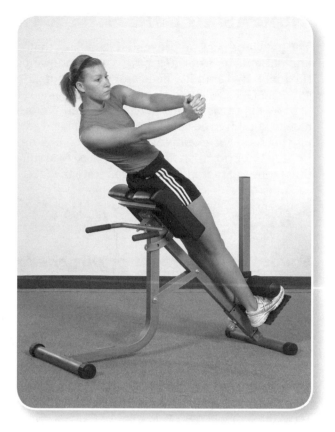

Russian Twist on a Physioball

Starting position: Supine position on top of the physioball. The hips are in a neutral position, the knees are flexed to 90°, and the feet are flat on the ground.

Movement: The client extends the arms above the chest and places the hands together. The client then rotates the arms to each side, holds the position for 1 to 2 seconds, then returns to the starting position. This exercise should be performed to both sides.

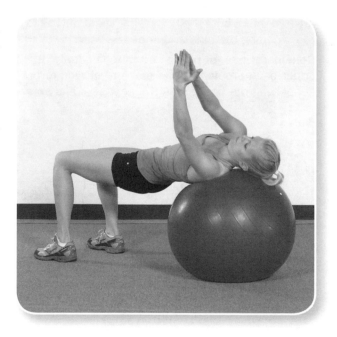

INCREASING CORE STRENGTH

The previous section presented exercises that are traditionally prescribed to clients and patients in order to improve core endurance capacity. Those exercises will meet the functional stability needs for most clients. However, the addition of strengthening exercises for the muscles of the core is necessary for athletes, manual laborers, and high-level fitness clients. These competitive or industrial athletes not only must be able to stabilize the spine but also must have adequate strength to perform functional movements. For example, a laborer who lifts heavy boxes all day long not only must be able to perform an abdominal brace to stabilize the spine but also must be able to utilize the correct muscles to generate the force needed to lift a heavy object.

Core Strength Exercises

Squat With a Barbells or Dumbbells

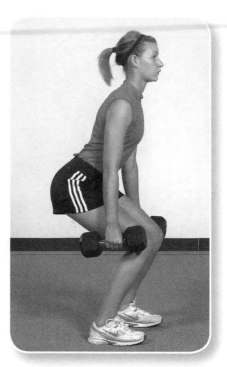

Starting position: Standing with the feet shoulder-width apart. When performing the squat with a barbell, the client holds a bar across the upper back; the bar should be resting on either the trapezius muscle or the trapezius and deltoids. When using dumbbells, the weights should be held at the sides of the body. If a barbell is used, a spotter should assist the client.

Movement: The client lowers her body by bending the hips and knees. The motion should be initiated by extending the hips back (posteriorly). The knees should not fall in front of the feet. The client squats, lowering herself to a position of almost full hip and knee flexion; the thighs should be parallel to the floor. The client must maintain a neutral spine posture throughout the squat. The client returns to the starting position by extending the hips and knees.

Considerations for rehab and fitness clients: If the client has neck or upper back problems, she may be allowed to perform a front squat, supporting the bar across the pectorals and anterior deltoid.

Romanian Deadlift

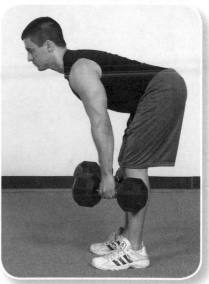

The Romanian deadlift strengthens the hamstrings and challenges the client's ability to stabilize the trunk.

Starting position: Standing with the feet hip-width apart while holding a pair of dumbbells (or a bar) a little wider than shoulder-width apart. The knees should be slightly bent, and the spine should be in a neutral posture.

Movement: The client lowers the bar toward the floor by shifting the hips back (posteriorly) until he feels a stretch in the hamstrings. The spine should not flex. The client returns to the starting position by contracting the hamstrings and pulling the dumbbells or bar toward the starting position.

Pull-Up

The pull-up exercise (also known as the chin-up) can be performed to improve general back strength as well as core stability (via the latissimus dorsi; see chapter 2). As with the lat pull-down exercise, various techniques are used for the pull-up.

Starting position: Holding the pull-up bar with the forearms in a pronated position (overhand grip). You may also want to have clients use other grips, such as the underhand grip.

Movement: The client inhales while pulling the body toward the bar. The client then slowly lowers the body to the starting position.

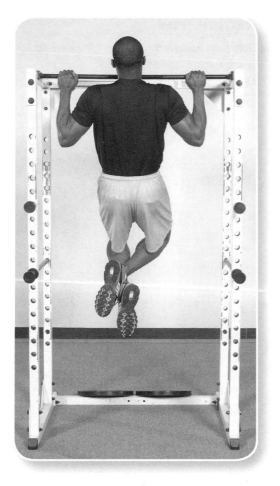

Lat Pull-Down

Starting position: Seated at the lat machine, facing the machine. The client should grasp the bar with a wide overhand grip.

Movement: The client pulls the bar toward the chest while squeezing the shoulder blades together and down toward the lower back.

Considerations for rehab and fitness clients: Some people advocate pulling the bar behind the neck instead of pulling it toward the chest. Care should be taken with this exercise, especially with clients who have a history of shoulder problems or instability.

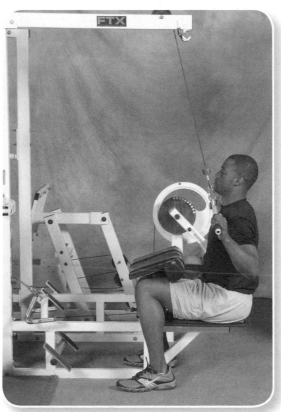

Seated Row

Starting position: Seated with a neutral spine posture while gripping the bar or handles

Movement: The client pulls the bar or handles toward the abdomen. Cue the client to squeeze the shoulder blades together and down toward the low back while he extends the upper arms to a position in line with the body.

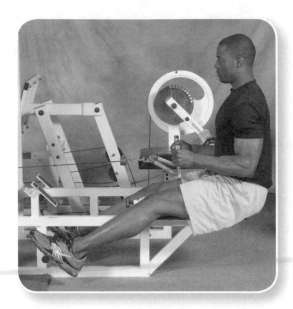

Cable Diagonal Patterns

Starting position: Standing perpendicular to the pulley machine. The handle is positioned either high or low on the machine. The client holds the cable handle in both hands.

Movement: The client performs a diagonal motion across his body in either a low-to-high or high-to-low direction. This exercise may also be performed with resistance tubing.

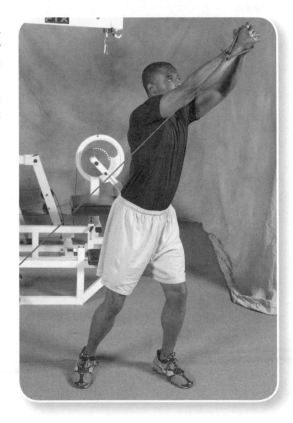

Lunge

This functional exercise strengthens the lower extremities and enhances core stability.

Starting position: Standing with the hips shoulder-width apart

Movement: The client steps (lunges) forward, flexing the lead hip and knee. The lead knee should be in alignment with the hip and foot, and the thigh should be parallel (or almost parallel) to the ground. The body is lowered toward the floor to the point where the trailing knee almost contacts the ground. The client then reverses the movement, returning to the starting position. The client repeats the lunging sequence with the opposite leg stepping forward.

Key tips: Cue the client to maintain ideal posture of the pelvis and low back. Observe the entire kinetic chain for technique errors.

Variation: A walking lunge may be performed by repeating alternating lunging sequences with a forward progression.

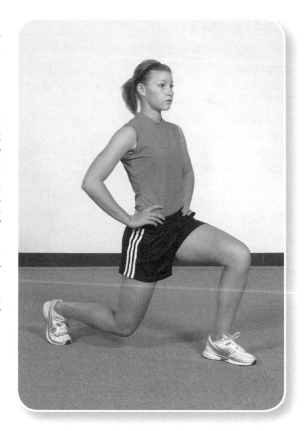

Lunge Twist

Starting position: Same as the lunge

Movement: When performing the lunge, the client rotates the trunk toward the side of the rear (trailing) leg. The client returns to the starting position and repeats to the opposite side.

Variation: The client can use a stick to help maintain balance.

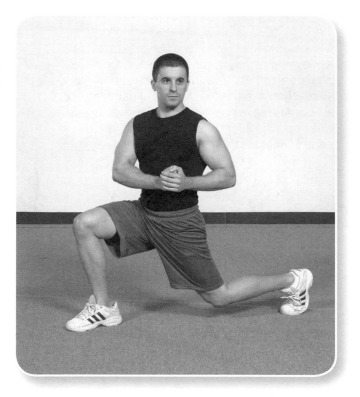

Backward Lunge

Starting position: Same as the forward lunge

Movement: The client performs a lunge that looks exactly the same as the traditional lunge except the trailing leg steps backward.

Variation: The backward lunge may also be performed by resting the trailing leg on a physioball. To perform the backward lunge, the client extends the hip, rolling the ball backward.

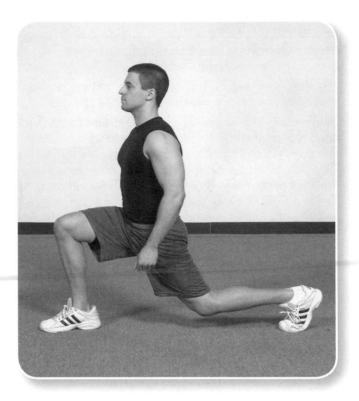

Lateral Lunge

Starting position: Standing with the hips shoulder-width apart

Movement: The client steps (lunges) to the side while keeping the feet pointed straight ahead. While performing the lateral lunge, the client should squat (sitting back) toward the floor. The stationary leg is passively abducted during the exercise. The client should keep the spine in a neutral posture throughout the exercise.

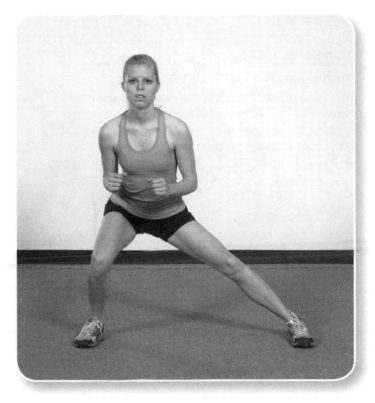

Lunge With Ball Rotation

Starting position: The client and a partner stand side by side, up to 3 feet (90 cm) apart and facing the same direction.

Movement: Both partners perform a walking lunge simultaneously. As the lunge is performed, the partner who is holding the ball rotates toward the other individual, handing her the ball. The walking lunge is repeated, and the partners take turns rotating and handing the ball to the other partner.

Variation: The lunge may also be performed without a partner. The client assumes the starting position by holding the ball in front of her body. As the client lunges, she rotates the ball to the side.

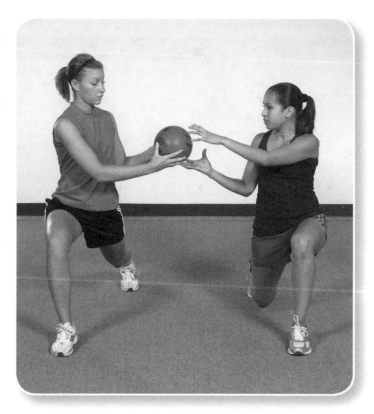

Chu's Lunge Series for Athletes

Don Chu, PhD, PT, is a leading authority in sports training and rehabilitation. He has been credited as a key proponent of plyometric exercises, helping to popularize this form of training in the United States (Chu and Cordier 2000). Dr. Chu promotes a specific lunge exercise sequence designed for athletes (personal communication, 2006). This sequence incorporates four lunging movements. The series consists of a forward lunge, a backward lunge, a lateral lunge, and a diagonal lunge 45° from a horizontal axis. Chu recommends having the athlete perform 10 repetitions of each exercise for a grand total of 80 reps!

SUMMARY

This chapter has presented a series of exercises designed to improve core endurance and strength. Remember to consider the client's fitness level when prescribing core exercises. Failure to prescribe the correct exercises will limit the effectiveness of the training program and may even contribute to injury. The data you collect from the physical assessment will help to guide your exercise selection. If in doubt, start a client at the basic level, progressing the client as soon as he demonstrates mastery of those exercises.

Table 6.2 Exercises That Train Specific Muscles of the Core

Muscles	Basic	Intermediate	Advanced	Strengthening
Trapezius	1. Straight-arm pull-down	1. Quadruped opposite arm and leg raise 2. Front plank with arm or leg extension 3. Front plank with opposite arm and leg extension	1. Hang twist	1. Pull-up 2. Seated row
Latissimus dorsi	1. Straight-arm pull-down	N/A	1. Hang twist	1. Lat pull-down
Erector spinae	1. Finding neutral spine in quadruped 2. Quadruped position with arm raise 3. Quadruped position with leg extension 4. Straight-arm pull-down 5. Wall lean 6. Cable side steps	1. Quadruped opposite arm and leg raise 2. Bridging with a march 3. Bridging with leg extension 4. Front plank 5. Front plank with arm or leg extension 6. Front plank with opposite arm and leg extension 7. Bridging with a physioball	1. Bridge and crunch exercise 2. Prone twist 3. Three-point plank with upper extremity exercise 4. Roman twist 5. Roman chair 6. Russian twist 7. Russian twist on a physioball	1. Romanian deadlift 2. Cable diagonal patterns
Transversospinalis muscle group	1. Straight-arm pull-down 2. Wall lean 3. Cable side steps	1. Quadruped opposite arm and leg raise 2. Bridging with a march 3. Bridging with leg extension 4. Front plank 5. Front plank with arm or leg extension 6. Front plank with opposite arm and leg extension 7. Bridging with a physioball	1. Bridge and crunch exercise 2. Prone twist 3. Three-point plank with upper extremity exercise 4. Roman twist 5. Roman chair 6. Russian twist 7. Russian twist on a physioball	1. Romanian deadlift 2. Cable diagonal patterns
Rectus abdominis	1. Crunch 2. Front plank with knee supports	1. Side bridge 2. Front plank 3. Front plank with arm or leg extension 4. Front plank with opposite arm and leg extension 5. Reverse crunch 6. Knee tuck on a physioball	1. Jackknife on the physioball 2. Hang twist 3. Prone twist 4. V ups 5. Leg raise 6. Roman twist 7. Russian twist	N/A
Transversus abdominis	1. Side bridge (beginner)	1. Side bridge	1. Jackknife on the physioball 2. Hang twist 3. Prone twist 4. V-ups 5. Leg raise 6. Roman twist 7. Russian twist	N/A

Muscles	Basic	Intermediate	Advanced	Strengthening
External oblique	1. Crunch 2. Front plank with knee supports	1. Front plank 2. Front plank with arm or leg extension 3. Front plank with opposite arm and leg extension 4. Crunch on the physioball 5. Ball plank twists	1. Jackknife on the physioball 2. Hang twist 3. Prone twist 4. V-ups 5. Leg raise 6. Roman twist 7. Russian twist	N/A
Internal oblique	1. Crunch 2. Front plank with knee supports	1. Front plank 2. Front plank with arm or leg extension 3. Front plank with opposite arm and leg extension 4. Crunch on the physioball 5. Ball plank twists	1. Jackknife on the physioball 2. Hang twist 3. Prone twist 4. V-ups 5. Leg raise 6. Roman twist 7. Russian twist	N/A
Hip flexors (iliacus and psoas major)	N/A	1. Knee tuck on a physioball	1. Hang twist 2. V-ups 3. Leg raise 4. Side bridge with hip flexion	N/A
Gluteus maximus	1. Prone hip extension 2. Bridging	1. Bridging with a march 2. Bridging with leg extension 3. Front plank with arm or leg extension 4. Front plank with opposite arm and leg extension	1. Inverted hamstring	1. Squat
Gluteus medius	1. Clamshell 2. Side-lying straight leg raise	1. Side bridge 2. Physioball leg raise	1. Side-lying bilateral leg raise 2. Side bridge with hip abduction 3. Side bridge with shoulder external rotation 4. Lunges	1. Squat
Gluteus minimus	1. Clamshell 2. Side-lying straight leg raise	1. Side bridge 2. Physioball leg raise	1. Side-lying bilateral leg raise 2. Side bridge with hip abduction 3. Side bridge with shoulder external rotation 4. Lunges	1. Squat

(continued)

Table 6.2 *(continued)*

Muscles	Basic	Intermediate	Advanced	Strengthening
Tensor fasciae latae	1. Clamshell 2. Side-lying straight leg raise	1. Side bridge	1. Side-lying bilateral leg raise 2. Side bridge with hip abduction 3. Side bridge with shoulder external rotation 4. Side bridge with hip flexion 5. Lunges	1. Squat
Piriformis	1. Clamshell	1. Ball plank twists	N/A	N/A
Hip external rotators	1. Clamshell 2. Side-lying straight leg raise	1. Standing torso rotation 2. Standing high-low torso rotations 3. Hip crossovers 4. Ball plank twists	1. Prone twist	N/A
Hip internal rotators	1. Side-lying straight leg raise	1. Ball plank twists	1. Prone twist	N/A

7

Core Flexibility

People need a certain degree of flexibility in order to perform their jobs and other activities of daily living. For example, a mover needs sufficient hip, knee, and ankle flexibility (combined with the ability to stabilize the spine) so that he can squat safely when lifting furniture. If the mover's flexibility is limited at any one joint, the mover will likely perform the lift with poor body mechanics, potentially increasing the risk of injury to that joint or an adjacent one. A golfer with poor core flexibility may be unable to optimally rotate her trunk during the backswing. This lack of flexibility will prevent the golfer from maximizing her club head speed during the downswing.

Stretching exercises should be prescribed to address a client's limited or poor flexibility. Additional benefits attributed to stretching include increasing relaxation, reducing stress, decreasing muscular tension, and maintaining or improving posture. Stretching may also decrease low back pain, relieve symptoms associated with muscular cramps or muscular soreness, and help prevent injuries (Alter 2004).

Flexibility exercises should be included in the training programs one designs for fitness clients, athletes, or patients. There are a variety of stretching techniques that may be prescribed. The challenge is to choose the most appropriate stretching technique for each client. When selecting exercises for a stretching program, one must consider the goal of the stretching program. Is it to

- increase flexibility,
- enhance athletic performance,
- reduce the risk of injury,
- rehabilitate a patient after an injury,

or some combination of these? The science behind flexibility is continually evolving. What may be believed to be true today may not be true tomorrow. Therefore, one must stay abreast of the trends and advances reported in the research literature.

The purpose of this chapter is to review stretching methodology, introduce an evidence-based approach to program design, and provide numerous flexibility exercises and sample programs that address the core.

WHAT IS FLEXIBILITY?

Any discussion of flexibility should begin with a review of terminology. Fitness professionals should know the meaning of the terms *range of motion* and *flexibility,* understand the modes of stretching, and recognize the indications and contraindications associated with prescribing a client a stretching program.

Range of motion (ROM) refers to the amount of motion available at a joint. Medical professionals typically measure ROM in degrees using a tool known as a **goniometer.** Fitness professionals typically identify a client's ROM limitations through observation of functional movement patterns and hands-on assessments. ROM is often described in one of two ways: **active range of motion (AROM)** or **passive range of motion (PROM).**

Flexibility relates to a person's ability to move through an available ROM. Flexibility is divided into two categories: static and dynamic (Holcomb 2000; Jeffreys 2008). **Static flexibility** refers to the ROM that can be demonstrated at a joint without any muscular contraction. Thus, rehabilitation professionals often refer to static flexibility as passive range of motion (PROM). **Dynamic flexibility** is the ROM demonstrated by a client when performing any active motion. This type of flexibility, also known as active range of motion, requires muscular activity. It is not unusual for a person's dynamic flexibility to be less than his static flexibility.

Some people may present with abnormal or excessive range of motion. When assessing a client's functional abilities, you may be able to determine whether the client demonstrates either excessive motion (**hypermobile**) or restricted motion (**hypomobile**). Hypermobility refers to ROM at a joint beyond accepted "normal" values (Alter 2004). For example, normal ROM for knee extension is 0°, but many females demonstrate excessive knee hyperextension of 10 to 20°. Using the Beighton score may help identify clients who are hypermobile (Boyle et al. 2003). A client is considered hypermobile if she scores at least five out of a possible nine points on the following tests:

- Score one point if the client can bend at the waist and place both hands flat on the floor while keeping her knees straight.
- Score one point for *each* knee that can bend into hyperextension.
- Score one point for *each* elbow that can hyperextend past neutral.
- Score one point for *each* thumb that is able to bend backward to touch the forearm.
- Score one point for *each* little finger that is able to bend backward beyond 90°.

Not to be confused with joint hypermobility, joint **laxity** is the excessive play or movement created at the joint when a supporting ligamentous structure is stretched or injured. Ligamentous laxity in the knee (which may result from a tear of the anterior cruciate ligament, for example) may contribute to knee instability, especially if the surrounding muscles are unable to adequately provide backup support and stability. A client who is hypermobile may be able to demonstrate normal function, whereas a client with joint laxity may have impaired function and ultimately may require medical attention.

Hypomobility of a joint or group of joints may limit functional movement. Many individuals are hypomobile in the lumbar spine. Although hypomobility in one region may not hinder a client's ability to perform a functional movement, it may result in suboptimal movement patterns. Suboptimal patterns typically involve using compensatory movement strategies. For example, an individual who has poor hip strength might demonstrate excessive spinal flexion when performing a squat. If poor movement patterns are repeated over time, that person's joints may have an increased risk of injury.

CLASSIFICATIONS OF STRETCHING

The four primary modes of stretching are static, dynamic, ballistic, and proprioceptive neuromuscular facilitation (PNF). All of these techniques can improve a client's flexibility; however, fitness professionals must understand when a particular mode should be used. This section provides a description and illustration of each technique, along with sample clinical suggestions and potential contraindications.

Static Stretching

A static stretch is a slow, controlled movement that lengthens a muscle or group of muscles for a sustained period of time (Holcomb 2000; Woods et al. 2007; Jeffreys 2008). To correctly perform a static stretch, clients should stretch to the position in which they feel a strong, yet comfortable, "stretching" sensation (or an increase in muscular tension) without experiencing pain.

Static stretching has been found to increase static flexibility and range of motion, thus potentially benefiting both healthy clients and injured patients (Alter 2004). A static stretching routine can help promote relaxation, reduce a client's stress level, decrease muscle soreness, and improve flexibility. Static stretching can be performed anywhere and anytime, and it can usually be performed without the assistance of a partner or an apparatus.

How long should a static stretch be held in order to achieve improved flexibility and range of motion? How many repetitions per stretch are necessary? When is the optimal time to do static stretching?

The literature is full of studies that compare the changes in flexibility that result from various hold times (e.g., 15 seconds versus 30 seconds, 5 seconds versus 60 seconds, and so on). On average, a static stretch should be held for a minimum of 30 seconds (Decoster et al. 2005; Bandy et al. 1994). The literature appears to lack studies regarding how many reps a person should perform per muscle group per training session. The clinical experience from a variety of professionals suggests that for a client to achieve flexibility improvements, the client should stretch the targeted muscle or muscle group for one or more reps on a daily basis. The client must be prepared to regularly perform these exercises in order to receive any benefit. It may take many weeks of daily stretching for a client to experience flexibility gains.

A static stretching routine should be performed at the end of the client's resistance training program or as part of a separate stretching session.

Some strength coaches and athletic trainers will have their athletes perform static stretches prior to practice or competition. The reported rationale for using static stretches as part of a warm-up routine is that it "prepares the muscles" for competition and helps to reduce the risk of injury (Alter 2004). Those who are opposed to athletes performing static stretching exercises prior to practice or competition contend that static stretching does not replicate the dynamic movements required for sports. Current research also challenges the use of static stretching immediately before performance (Stone et al. 2006; Yamaguchi et al. 2006). For example, researchers found that the use of static stretching actually decreased vertical jump performance when the stretching occurred immediately before the jump (Bradley et al. 2007).

Static stretching techniques may be useful in clinical rehabilitation settings. During the acute (immediately after an injury) or subacute phases of an injury, static stretching may allow the patient to safely improve range of motion, whereas active forms of stretching may exacerbate symptoms. Having a patient perform static stretches may also provide the additional benefits of reducing muscular soreness, decreasing pain, and inducing general relaxation.

Table 7.1 shows indications and contraindications for static stretching. The sidebar shows a sample static stretching routine for the core.

Table 7.1   Indications, Contraindications, and Dosing for Static Stretching

Indications	Contraindications	Recommended number of reps	Duration
To increase flexibility, induce relaxation, decrease pain, and decrease muscle soreness	When movement is not indicated (e.g., specific medical conditions, surgery, or fracture); if stretching increases pain; immediately before sport or training	1 or more repetitions (clinical examples suggest at least 2 reps per muscle or muscle group)	30-second holds

---

Sample Static Stretching Routine for the Core

Repetitions: 2 repetitions of each stretch

Duration: 30-second hold for each stretch

Rest: 10 to 20 seconds of rest between each repetition (photos and descriptions for each stretch are presented at the end of the chapter)

Supine Position
- Knee to chest stretch (both legs)
- Hamstring stretch
- Piriformis stretch

Kneeling Position
- Hip flexor stretch

Prone Position
- Cobra pose
- Prayer stretch
- Prayer stretch with side bend

Dynamic Stretching

Dynamic stretching incorporates sport-specific movements in order to enhance functional flexibility. Some people classify dynamic stretching as a type of ballistic stretching because both forms of stretching involve movement (Alter 2004; Woods et al. 2007). However, dynamic stretching does not include the bouncing or bobbing movements characteristic of ballistic stretching. Instead, dynamic stretching emphasizes sport-specific movement patterns (Holcomb 2000; Jeffreys 2008). Examples of dynamic stretches include the forward lunge, the backward (reverse) lunge, and high-knee marching.

Dynamic stretching has recently gained popularity; a growing body of evidence supports the use of dynamic stretching to warm up athletes or clients before a sport or training session (Hendrick 2000; Little and Williams 2006; Faigenbaum et al. 2005; Yamaguchi et al. 2006; Hewett et al. 1999). Table 7.2 shows indications and contraindications for dynamic stretching, and a sample dynamic warm-up routine is shown in the sidebar.

Table 7.2 Indications, Contraindications, and Dosing for Dynamic Stretching

Indications	Contraindications	Recommended number of reps	Duration
To increase functional flexibility and to metabolically prepare the client or athlete for training or sport	When active movements are not indicated (e.g., specific medical conditions, surgery, fracture)	Perform 6 to 7 dynamic movements	The athlete should perform each dynamic movement for approximately 1 to 2 minutes per dynamic drill for a total of 10 or more minutes

Ballistic Stretching

A ballistic stretch involves the use of active movements that incorporate bouncing or bobbing. Ballistic stretching differs from static stretching in that the end position is not held for a set period of time (Holcomb 2000; Alter 2004; Jeffreys 2008). Ballistic stretching is used predominately as a modality to warm up or prepare the athlete for sport (Bradley et al. 2007). Bending forward toward the floor and then repetitively

Sample Dynamic Warm-Up Routine

A dynamic stretching routine should consist of activities that metabolically prepare the client or athlete for more intense forms of exercise or activity. You should also choose activities that closely replicate the functional or sport-specific movement patterns applicable for the client. The sidebar presents a sample dynamic stretching routine for a basketball player. This warm-up routine is performed before practice or competition.

Sample Dynamic Stretching Routine for Basketball

The athlete begins by jogging 5 laps around the court.

The athlete performs each of the following dynamic activities for 1 or 2 widths of the basketball court. The entire routine should last approximately 10 minutes.

Crossover toe touch	Walking side lunge
Walking lunge	Walking on heels
Walking reverse lunge	Walking on toes

bouncing in an effort to increase hamstring flexibility is a classic example of a ballistic stretch.

Proponents of ballistic stretching argue that it helps develop dynamic flexibility (Alter 2004; Woolstenhulme et al. 2006). Many people reject the use of ballistic stretching because of a purported risk of injury. Is ballistic stretching dangerous? Many fitness professionals discount the potential effectiveness of this form of stretching based on the specific client or patient populations they train or treat. However, there is a lack of research evidence to support the claim that ballistic stretching may harm a client. To the contrary, studies have demonstrated that in some cases ballistic stretching may be as effective as (or preferable to) other modes of stretching (Beedle and Mann 2007; Bradley et al. 2007). Caution should be applied if an athlete or client has had a previous injury that may be aggravated by this form of stretching. For example, an athlete who has had a history of low back pain due to a lumbar disk injury may increase his risk of reinjury when performing a ballistic toe touching movement. Table 7.3 lists indications and contraindications for ballistic stretching.

Table 7.3 Indications, Contraindications, and Dosing for Ballistic Stretching

Indications	Contraindications	Recommended number of reps	Duration
To warm up before sport or exercise	Rehab patients; individuals with a previous herniated disc, a history of recurrent low back pain, or a recent history of muscle strains	15 ballistic stretches during a 30-second period (Beedle and Mann 2007)	One 30-second set per muscle group (Beedle and Mann 2007)

Proprioceptive Neuromuscular Facilitation (PNF) Stretching

PNF stretching is performed with a partner and involves both passive movements and active muscle actions (Alter 2004; Holcomb 2000). A benefit of using PNF stretching is that it may cause immediate gains in flexibility. The effectiveness of PNF stretching in making lasting flexibility improvements is less clear. Table 7.4 lists indications and contraindications for PNF stretching. To perform most PNF stretching techniques, a person must have the assistance of a partner. This limits the overall utility of PNF stretching. The main PNF techniques are hold-relax, agonist contraction, contract relax, and hold-relax with agonist contraction. An example of each technique is provided in the following sections. These techniques can be applied to almost any muscle or muscle group in the body. The hamstrings are used as a reference point in each of the following examples.

Table 7.4 Indications, Contraindications, and Dosing for PNF Stretching

Indications	Contraindications	Recommended number of reps	Duration
To warm up before sport or exercise and to increase flexibility in fitness and rehab clients	When movement is not indicated	2 to 4 repetitions per muscle or muscle group	See duration periods for each technique in the following sections.

Hold-Relax (HR)

To start, have the client assume a supine position on a floor or mat. Next, you should passively stretch the client's hamstrings to the point that a strong stretch is experienced by the client. This initial end position should be held for up to 10 seconds. Then ask the client to isometrically contract the hamstrings for up to 10 seconds while you apply a matching force in the opposite direction. Next, the client relaxes the contraction followed immediately by you passively stretching the muscle beyond the initial stretch position. Hold this stretch for 30 seconds. Perform 2 to 4 repetitions per muscle or muscle group.

Agonist Contraction

To start, have the client assume a supine position on a floor or mat. Next, perform the passive stretch of the client's hamstring muscle group as in the previous technique, holding for 10 seconds. After the 10-second hold, instruct the client to contract the agonist muscle group (in this case, the hip flexors) while you provide resistance to hip flexion for 6 to 10 seconds. After the isometric hip flexion, you should again passively flex the client at the hip (while the knee remains extended) in order to stretch the hamstrings. Hold the stretch for 30 seconds. Perform 2 to 4 agonist contractions per muscle or muscle group.

Contract Relax

To apply the contract relax stretch to the hamstrings, have the client assume a supine position on the floor or on a mat. Next, passively stretch the client's hamstrings to the point that he experiences a strong stretch. Hold this position for up to 10 seconds. Next, instruct the client to contract his hamstrings, extending his hip through the entire range of motion while you provide some resistance to the motion. At the end of hip extension immediately passively stretch the client's hamstrings beyond the initial stretch position. Hold this stretch for 30 seconds. Perform 2 to 4 repetitions per muscle or muscle group.

Hold-Relax With Agonist Contraction

This technique combines the hold-relax technique with an additional agonist contraction. After the client performs the isometric contraction of the hamstrings (10 seconds), the client should allow the hamstrings to relax. The client should then immediately begin to actively flex the hip (the agonist) against resistance. After 6 to 10 seconds, the client should relax all muscle groups, which will allow you to further stretch the hamstrings. Repeat this technique for 2 to 4 repetitions to maximize muscular flexibility.

USE OF FOAM ROLLS IN STRETCHING

A popular exercise trend in sports medicine clinics and fitness training centers is to incorporate the use of a foam roller when performing flexibility exercises. Stretching techniques performed in conjunction with a foam roll have been called self-myofascial-release stretching (SMFR) (Clark and Russell 2002). Proponents of SMFR claim that it helps decrease soft-tissue pain, improves muscular balance between agonists and antagonists, and enhances function. This technique is believed to increase soft-tissue extensibility by finding "hot spots" (although not well defined, hot spots are likely trigger points that have developed in the muscle; see chapter 2) and "releasing" these areas of increased sensitivity through direct pressure (Kaltenborn 2006). It has been proposed that when the client applies pressure to a hot spot, a reflexive relaxation of the muscle will occur (Clark and Russell 2002).

For many clients, performing stretching exercises with a foam roller will be a new experience. When prescribing a stretching program that incorporates a foam roller, you will likely need to provide a physical demonstration in addition to the verbal instructions for each stretching position. Keep the following points in mind when teaching your client how to stretch with a foam roller:

- Instruct the client to move or "roll over" the muscle or muscle group at a rate of 1 inch (2.5 cm) per second (Clark and Russell 2002; Kaltenborn 2006).
- Explain to the client that there may be areas within the muscle that feel tender (the hot spot).
- When a hot spot is found, instruct the client to hold that position, maintaining pressure on that point for 30 to 60 seconds (Clark and Russell 2002; Kaltenborn 2006).
- Encourage the client to maintain this position, even in the presence of minor to moderate pain.
- If the client experiences pain that is unbearable, instruct the client to try to unload just enough pressure in the "hold" position to make it tolerable.

Despite the popularity of this form of stretching, the actual benefits are unknown. There is a lack of research literature relating to the efficacy of this form of stretching. Research has not determined whether SMFR (foam roller stretching) is superior to traditional forms of stretching when it comes to improving flexibility. Also, the short- and long-term effectiveness of the SMFR technique in relieving pain is not known. SMFR is similar to sport massage in that numerous claims regarding its effectiveness abound, but evidence supporting these claims is limited or altogether absent (Barlow et al. 2004; Hopper et al. 2005; Brumitt 2008).

The following section presents a few techniques that incorporate the use of a foam roll. If you choose to include the foam roll in a client's training program, do so in conjunction with other traditional forms of stretching.

STRETCHES

This section presents static, dynamic, PNF, and foam roll stretching techniques for many of the muscles of the core. The stretches are organized by muscle group.

Stretching the Hamstrings

Static Stretching Techniques for the Hamstrings

Numerous static stretching techniques have been developed for the hamstring muscle group. The variety of techniques allows strength training professionals to pick the most suitable position for each client.

Starting Position 1

Starting position: The client lies on his back, grabbing the back of his knee with both hands.

Movement: The client actively flexes the hip to 90°. While maintaining this position, the client extends (straightens) the knee until he feels a strong stretch in the hamstrings.

Variations for position 1: If the client is unable to grab the knee and support the position with both hands (e.g., because of obesity or poor upper body strength), the client may use a towel or stretch band to assist.

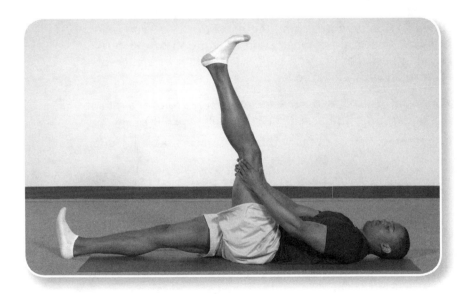

Starting Position 2

Starting position: The client lies supine in a doorway.

Movement: The client places a foot on the door frame. While keeping his knee extended, the client slides his body closer to the door. The stretch position is held once he feels a strong stretch in the hamstrings.

Starting position 3

Starting position: The client is sitting with one or both legs straight.

Movement: The client reaches for the toes while maintaining a neutral spine. The stretch position is held once she feels a strong stretch in the hamstrings. Many clients have a tendency to bend or flex from the thoracic and lumbar spine instead of bending at the hips.

Starting position 4

Starting position: While standing, the client places a foot on a small step.

Movement: The client leans forward toward the foot on the step (as if attempting to touch her toes) by flexing at the hips. The stretch position is held once she feels a strong stretch in the hamstrings. Again, the client should maintain a neutral spine and an extended knee.

Dynamic Stretching Techniques for the Hamstrings

When a person is performing a dynamic stretch, many muscles will be trained. Therefore, this form of stretching is effective for metabolically warming up the body before exercise or sport.

Crossover Toe Touch

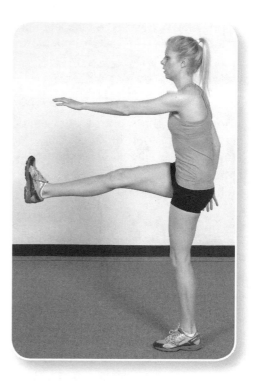

Starting position: The client is standing with the feet shoulder-width apart.

Movement: The client kicks a leg straight out in front of the body, attempting to touch the foot by reaching with the opposite hand.

Muscles: This stretching exercise addresses the muscles of the trunk, the latissimus dorsi, the hip flexors, the gluteus maximus and medius, the rectus femoris, and the hamstrings. Specifically, when this exercise is performed, the hamstring and gluteals are stretched on the kicking leg, whereas the contralateral latissimus dorsi and trunk muscles are dynamically stretched.

Hand Walking

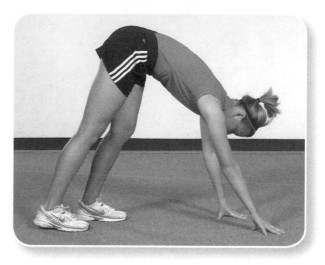

Starting position: The client assumes a position with both feet and both hands on the floor.

Movement: The client walks the hands away from the body while attempting to keep the legs straight and the feet on the ground. When the client can no longer hold this position, she then walks her feet towards the hands. This sequence is repeated through the desired distance.

Muscles: This stretching exercise addresses the muscles of the trunk, the hip extensors, the hip abductors, and the hamstrings. The lumbar extensors (erector spinae), the gluteus maximus and medius, and the hamstrings are stretched during this dynamic movement pattern.

Walking Lunge

Starting position: The client is standing with the hips shoulder-width apart.

Movement: The client steps (lunges) forward, flexing the lead hip and knee. The lead knee should be in alignment with the hip and foot, and the thigh should be parallel to the ground. The body is lowered toward the floor to the point where the trailing knee almost contacts the ground. The trailing leg is brought forward as the client assumes the standing position again. The lunging sequence is repeated with the opposite leg stepping forward. The client continues this pattern, performing the walking lunge for 1 to 2 minutes.

Muscles: This movement addresses the muscles of the trunk, the muscles of the hip, the quadriceps, and the hamstrings.

Variations: To increase the challenge for the abdominal muscles, the client should rotate to the side opposite the lead leg. For a greater challenge, the client may also hold a light medicine ball in his outstretched arms.

Walking Reverse Lunge

Starting position: Same as the forward lunge

Movement: The client performs a lunge that looks exactly the same as the traditional lunge except that the trailing leg starts the motion by stepping backward. The walking reverse lunge should be performed for 1 to 2 minutes.

Muscles: This movement addresses the muscles of the trunk, the muscles of the hip, the quadriceps, and the hamstrings.

PNF Stretching Techniques for the Hamstrings

Hold-Relax (HR)

- Have the client assume a supine position on a floor or mat.
- Passively stretch the client's hamstrings (the knee should remain extended) to the point that a strong stretch is experienced by the client. This initial end position should be held for up to 10 seconds.
- Ask the client to isometrically contract the hamstrings for up to 10 seconds while you apply a matching force in the opposite direction.
- When the client relaxes the contraction, you should immediately passively stretch the muscle beyond the initial stretch position. Hold this stretch for 30 seconds.
- Perform 2 to 4 repetitions per muscle or muscle group.

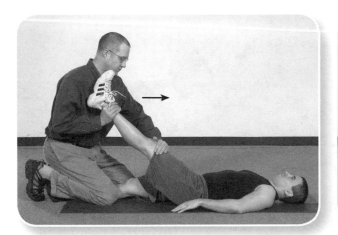

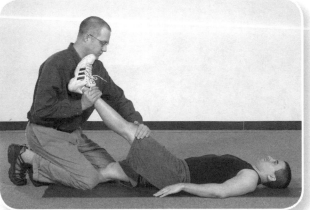

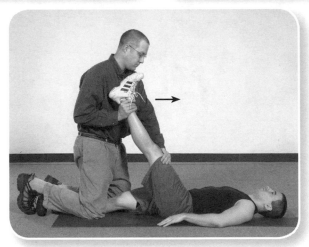

Agonist Contraction

- Have the client assume a supine position on a floor or mat.
- Passively stretch the client's hamstrings to the point that a strong stretch is experienced by the client. Hold this stretch for 10 seconds.
- After the 10-second hold, instruct the client to contract the hip flexors while you provide resistance to hip flexion for 6 to 10 seconds (second photo).
- After the isometric contraction (hip flexion), you should again passively flex the client at the hip in order to stretch the hamstrings. Hold the stretch for 30 seconds.
- Perform 2 to 4 agonist contractions per muscle or muscle group.

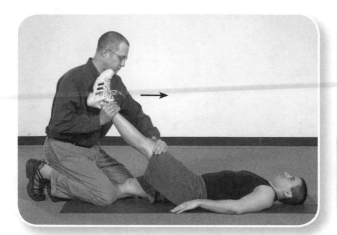
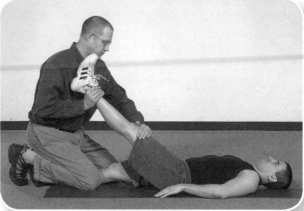
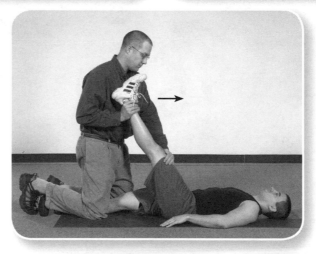

Contract Relax

- Have the client assume a supine position on the floor, mat, or table.
- Passively stretch the client's hamstrings to the point a strong stretch is experienced by the client. Hold this position for up to 10 seconds.
- Next, instruct the client to contract the hamstrings, extending the hip through the entire range of motion while you provide some resistance to the motion.
- At the end of hip extension immediately passively stretch the client's hamstrings beyond the initial stretch position. Hold this stretch for 30 seconds. Perform 2 to 4 repetitions per muscle or muscle group.

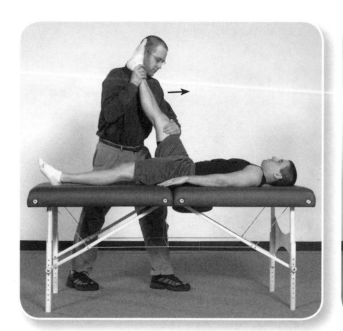
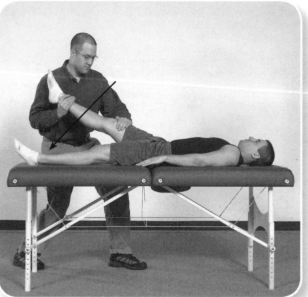
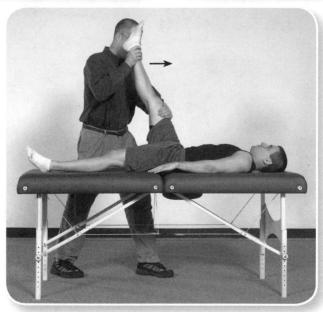

Hold-Relax With Agonist Contraction

This technique combines the hold-relax technique with an additional agonist contraction.

- Have the client assume a supine position on a floor or mat.
- Passively stretch the client's hamstrings to the point that a strong stretch is experienced by the client. Hold this stretch for 10 seconds.
- After the client performs the isometric contraction of the hamstrings (10 seconds), the client should allow the hamstrings to relax. The client should then immediately begin to actively flex his hip (the agonist) against resistance.
- After 6 to 10 seconds, the client should relax all muscle groups, which will allow you to further stretch the hamstrings. Hold the stretch for 30 seconds.
- Repeat this technique for 2 to 4 repetitions to maximize muscular flexibility.

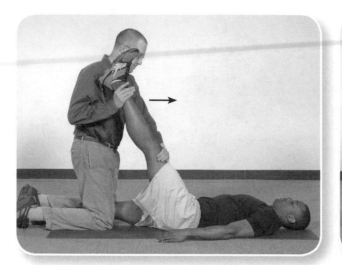

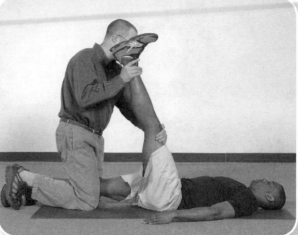

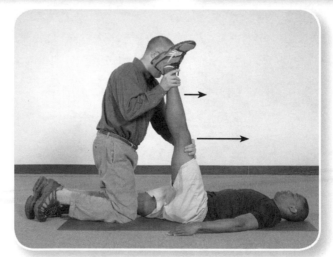

Foam Roll Application for the Hamstrings

Starting position: The client places the leg with the hamstrings to be stretched on top of the foam roll. She will then cross the opposite leg over, resting the opposite foot on top of the leg.

Movement: The client rolls over the leg along the length of the hamstrings.

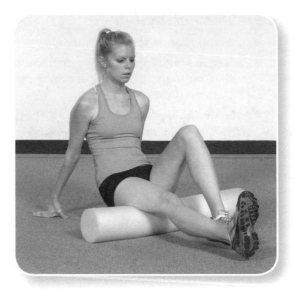

Stretching the Quadriceps

Static Stretching Technique for the Quadriceps

Starting position: The client is standing upright with one hand (the hand opposite the leg to be stretched) placed against a stable surface to help maintain balance.

Movement: The client bends (flexes) the knee toward the buttock, grabbing the foot. The client pulls the heel toward the buttocks and then holds this position. The spine and hip should be kept in a neutral position, and the knees should remain in the same plane.

Variations: This same stretch may be performed in a side-lying position. The strength training professional may be able to manually stretch the client's quadriceps when the client is in a prone position. To do this, grasp the ankle and slowly bend it toward the client's buttock. Hold the position for 30 seconds once the client notes that she is experiencing a strong stretch or when you notice the hip begin to lift off the table.

Dynamic Stretching Techniques for the Quadriceps

Walking lunge (see p. 98)

Walking reverse lunge (see p. 98)

PNF Stretching Techniques for the Quadriceps

Hold-Relax (HR)

- Have the client assume a prone position on a floor or mat.
- Grasp the client's ankle and then passively bend the client's knee (bringing the foot closer to the buttock).
- Stretch the client's quadriceps to the point that a strong stretch is experienced by the client. This initial end position should be held for up to 10 seconds.
- Ask the client to isometrically contract the quadriceps muscle for up to 10 seconds while you apply a matching force in the opposite direction.
- When the client relaxes the contraction, you should immediately passively stretch the muscle beyond the initial stretch position, bringing the foot closer to the buttock. Hold this stretch for 30 seconds.
- Perform 2 to 4 repetitions per muscle or muscle group.

Agonist Contraction

- Have the client assume a prone position on a floor or mat.
- Passively stretch the client's quadriceps (as previously described for the hold-relax technique) to the point that a strong stretch is experienced by the client. Hold this stretch for 10 seconds.
- After the 10-second hold, instruct the client to contract the hamstrings while you provide resistance to the knee flexing for 6 to 10 seconds.
- After the isometric hamstring contraction, you should again passively flex the client's knee in order to stretch the quadriceps. Hold the stretch for 30 seconds.
- Perform 2 to 4 agonist contractions per muscle or muscle group.

Hold-Relax With Agonist Contraction

- Have the client assume a prone position on a floor or mat.
- Passively stretch the client's quadriceps to the point that a strong stretch is experienced by the client. Hold this stretch for 10 seconds.
- After the client performs the isometric contraction of the quadriceps (10 seconds), the client should allow the quadriceps to relax. The client should then immediately begin to actively flex the hamstrings (the agonist) against resistance.
- After 6 to 10 seconds, the client should relax all muscle groups, which will allow you to further stretch the quadriceps. Hold this stretch for 30 seconds.
- Repeat this technique for 2 to 4 repetitions to maximize muscular flexibility.

Foam Roll Application for the Quadriceps

Starting position: The client assumes a prone position with the quadriceps placed on the foam roll; both forearms are supporting the upper body.

Movement: Using her upper body, the client rolls along the length of the quadriceps.

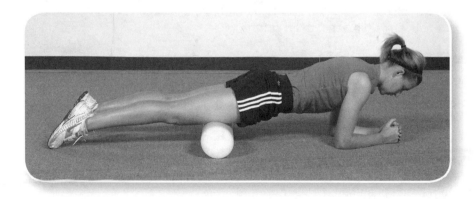

Stretching the Tensor Fasciae Latae (TFL) and the Iliotibial Band (ITB)

The tensor fasciae latae (TFL) muscle arises from the upper anterior portion of the pelvis, and it inserts into the iliotibial band (ITB). The ITB is a tendinous structure extending from the gluteus maximus and the tensor fasciae latae. The ITB inserts at the fibular head, the lateral patellar retinaculum, and Gerdy's tubercle on the lateral aspect of the tibia (Paluska 2005; Messier et al. 1995). Pain in this lateral region is common for certain types of athletes such as distance runners.

Irritation to the ITB (known as iliotibial band syndrome) has been a source of pain for those who ramp up their training mileage too quickly and those who train incorrectly. Treatment programs include stretching the ITB as a key component to a comprehensive rehabilitation program. The following set of stretches will address both the tensor fasciae latae and the iliotibial band.

Static Stretching Techniques for the TFL and ITB

Starting position: The client is standing near a wall and is using the arm closest to the wall to provide support. The leg closest to the wall is crossed behind the opposite leg.

Movement: To create the stretch, the client side bends the trunk away from the wall.

Variations: The client is positioned in the same starting pose. She brings her hands together above her head. To create the stretch, the client side bends to the side opposite the hip being stretched while keeping her arms extended overhead. Researchers found that this position provided the best pose for increasing ITB length (Fredericson et al. 2002).

Dynamic Stretching Techniques for the TFL and ITB

Trail Leg Walking

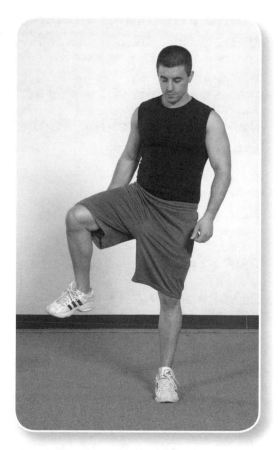

Starting position: The client assumes a standing position with the legs approximately shoulder-width apart.

Movement: The client first lifts the knee out to the side and then swings the foot to the front of the body to take the next step.

Muscles: This dynamic stretch addresses the hip flexors, the hip abductors, the hip external rotators, the TFL, and the quadriceps.

PNF Stretching Techniques for the TFL and ITB

See the PNF techniques for the hip external and internal rotators (p. 112).

Foam Roll Application for the Iliotibial Band

Starting position: The client assumes a side-lying position on the foam roll. The client flexes the hip of the top leg and positions it so that the foot can rest to the front of the bottom leg.

Movement: The client rolls his body the length of the upper leg (from the top of the pelvis to a point just below the knee joint).

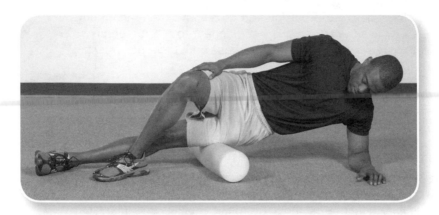

Stretching the Gluteus Maximus

Static Stretching Techniques for the Gluteus Maximus

Starting position: The client lies on the floor with both knees in a hook-lying position. One leg is crossed over the thigh of the other leg.

Movement: Using both hands, the client grabs behind the knee of the lower leg, pulling the legs toward the torso. The client then holds this position.

Dynamic Stretching Techniques for the Gluteus Maximus

Walking lunge (see p. 98)

Walking reverse lunge (see p. 98)

Crossover toe touch (see p. 97)

Hand walking (see p. 97)

PNF Stretching Techniques for the Gluteus Maximus

Hold-Relax (HR)

- Have the client assume a supine position on a floor or mat.
- Grasp the client's leg at the thigh and the lower leg.
- Lift the leg toward the chest, bending the hip and knee while rotating the hip. Bring the foot toward the midline until the client feels a strong stretch. This initial stretch position should be held for up to 10 seconds.

- Ask the client to isometrically contract the gluteus maximus (say "try to extend your leg" and "rotate your foot toward me") for up to 10 seconds while you apply a matching force in the opposite direction.
- When the client relaxes the contraction, you should immediately passively stretch the muscle beyond the initial stretch position. Hold this stretch for 30 seconds.
- Perform 2 to 4 repetitions per muscle or muscle group.

Agonist Contraction

- Have the client assume a supine position on a floor or mat.
- Grasp the client's leg at the thigh and the lower leg.
- Lift the leg toward the chest, bending the hip and knee while rotating the leg. Bring the foot toward the midline until the client feels a strong stretch. Hold this stretch for 10 seconds.
- After the 10-second hold, instruct the client to contract the hip flexors and hip internal rotators while you provide resistance to this movement for 6 to 10 seconds.
- After this isometric contraction, you should again passively flex and externally rotate the client's hip in order to stretch the gluteus maximus. Hold the stretch for 30 seconds.
- Perform 2 to 4 agonist contractions per muscle or muscle group.

Hold-Relax With Agonist Contraction

- Have the client assume a supine position on a floor or mat.
- Passively stretch the client's gluteus maximus to the point that a strong stretch is experienced by the client. Hold this stretch for 10 seconds.
- After the client performs the isometric contraction (10 seconds), the client should allow the gluteus maximus to relax. The client should then immediately begin to actively flex and internally rotate the hip (the agonist movement) against resistance.
- After 6 to 10 seconds, the client should relax all muscle groups, which will allow you to further stretch the gluteus maximus. Hold this stretch for 30 seconds.
- Repeat this technique for 2 to 4 repetitions to maximize muscular flexibility.

Foam Roll Application for the Gluteus Maximus

Starting position: The client is seated on the foam roll. By shifting weight to one side, the client can focus the stretch to one side of the buttock.

Movement: The client rolls from the upper hamstring across the buttock to the lower back.

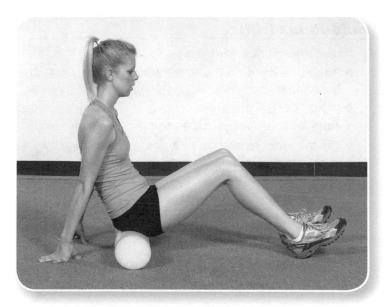

Stretching the Hip Flexors

Static Stretching Techniques for the Hip Flexors

Kneeling Hip Flexor Stretch

Starting position: The client assumes a lunge position with one foot positioned beyond the forward knee; the trailing knee is positioned on the floor.

Movement: The client shifts her body weight forward. The client will experience a stretch in the anterior hip and quadriceps of the trailing leg.

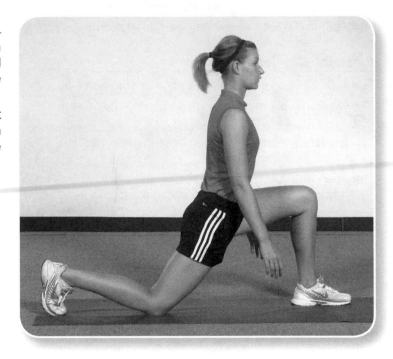

Dynamic Stretching Techniques for the Hip Flexors

Walking lunge (see p. 98)

Walking reverse lunge (see p. 98)

Crossover toe touch (see p. 97)

PNF Stretching Techniques for the Hip Flexors

Hold-Relax (HR)

- Have the client lie prone on a floor or mat.
- Place one hand on the client's low back and the other hand on the client's thigh (just above the knee).
- Gently stretch the anterior hip and anterior thigh by pulling the leg away from the surface. This initial stretch position should be held for up to 10 seconds.
- Ask the client to isometrically contract the hip flexors for up to 10 seconds while you apply a matching force in the opposite direction.
- When the client relaxes the contraction, you should immediately passively stretch the muscle beyond the initial stretch position. Hold this stretch for 30 seconds.
- Perform 2 to 4 repetitions per muscle or muscle group.

Agonist Contraction

- Have the client lie prone on a floor or mat.
- Place one hand on the client's low back and the other hand on the client's thigh (just above the knee).
- Gently stretch the anterior hip and anterior thigh by pulling the leg away from the surface. This initial stretch position should be held for up to 10 seconds.
- After the 10-second hold, instruct the client to contract the hip extensors (gluteus maximus) (say "try to lift your leg up higher without extending the spine") while you provide resistance to this movement (slide your hand from the front of the thigh to the back of the thigh) for 6 to 10 seconds.
- After this isometric contraction, you should again passively stretch the client, holding for 30 seconds.
- Perform 2 to 4 agonist contractions per muscle or muscle group.

Hold-Relax With Agonist Contraction

- Have the client lie prone on a floor or mat.
- Place one hand on the client's low back and the other hand on the client's thigh (just above the knee).
- Gently stretch the anterior hip and anterior thigh by pulling the leg away from the surface. This initial stretch position should be held for up to 10 seconds.
- After the client performs the isometric contraction (10 seconds), the client should allow the hip flexors to relax. The client should then immediately actively contract the hip extensors (the agonist) against resistance.
- After 6 to 10 seconds, the client should relax all muscle groups, which will allow you to further stretch the hip adductors. Hold this stretch for 30 seconds.
- Repeat this technique for 2 to 4 repetitions to maximize muscular flexibility.

Foam Roll Application for the Hip Adductors

Starting position: The client assumes a partially side-lying posture with the inner thigh of the leg to be stretched resting on the foam roll. The client should support himself with the hand of the side to be stretched (ipsilateral hand) and opposite (contralateral) forearm and elbow.

Movement: The client rolls his inner thigh along the foam roll from the inner hip to the knee.

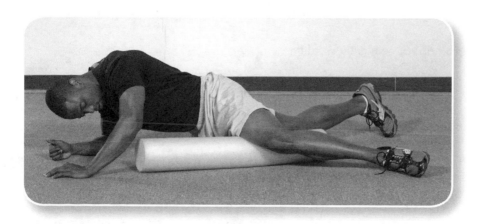

Stretching the Hip Adductors

The hip adductors arise from the pelvis and consist of the muscles of the inner thigh.

Static Stretching Techniques for the Hip Adductors

Supine Adductor Stretch

Starting position: The client lies in a supine position. The hips are externally rotated, and both feet are placed together.

Movement: The client allows both knees to lower toward the floor.

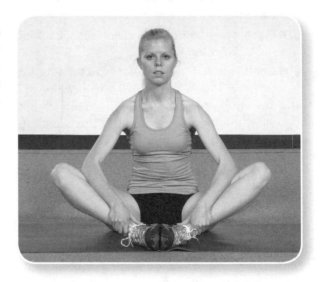

Sitting Groin Stretch

Starting position: The client is sitting on the floor with the soles of both feet together and drawn close to the body.

Movement: The client grasps the ankles with both hands and uses the elbows to press the knees toward the floor.

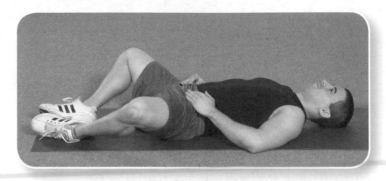

Kneeling Side Lunge

Starting position: The client kneels on the floor with one hip externally rotated in order to point the foot toward the side.

Movement: The client leans her body weight toward the supporting foot.

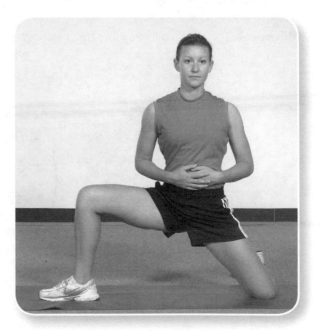

Dynamic Stretching Techniques for the Hip Adductors

Side Lunge Stretch

Starting position: The client stands with the feet shoulder-width apart and the hands on the hips. The feet are slightly externally rotated, helping to keep the foot, knee, and hip in alignment.

Movement: The client leans (lunges) toward one side. The client should hold this position for 30 seconds, experiencing a stretch on the inner thigh of the opposite leg. The client then brings the trailing leg toward the midline and returns to the starting position. The client should repeat this motion at least 2 times in one direction; then reverse directions and repeat at least 2 times in the other direction

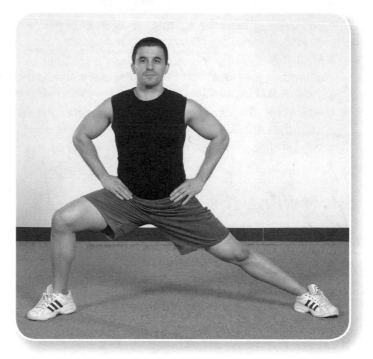

PNF Stretching Techniques for the Hip Adductors

Hold-Relax (HR)

- Have the client lie supine in a hook-lying position.
- Place your hands to the inside of each of the client's thighs at or just above the knee.
- Gently stretch the inner thigh by pushing each leg toward the floor until the client feels a strong stretch. This initial stretch position should be held for up to 10 seconds.
- Ask the client to isometrically contract the hip adductors for up to 10 seconds while you apply a matching force in the opposite direction.
- When the client relaxes the contraction, you should immediately passively stretch the muscle beyond the initial stretch position, increasing the hip adduction. Hold this stretch for 30 seconds.
- Perform 2 to 4 repetitions per muscle or muscle group.

Agonist Contraction

- Have the client lie supine in a hook-lying position.
- Place your hands to the inside of each of the client's thighs at or just above the knee.
- Gently stretch the inner thigh by pushing each leg toward the floor until the client feels a strong stretch. Hold the stretch for 10 seconds.
- After the 10-second hold, instruct the client to contract the lateral hip muscles (say "try to push your knees to the floor") while you provide resistance to this movement (place your hands on the lateral side of each knee) for 6 to 10 seconds.
- After this isometric contraction, you should again passively adduct the client's hip in order to stretch the inner thigh. Hold the stretch for 30 seconds.
- Perform 2 to 4 agonist contractions per muscle or muscle group.

Hold-Relax With Agonist Contraction

- Have the client lie supine in a hook-lying position.
- Passively stretch the client's hip adductors (inner thigh) to the point that a strong stretch is experienced by the client. Hold this stretch for 10 seconds.
- After the client performs the isometric contraction (10 seconds), the client should allow the hip adductors to relax. The client should then immediately actively contract the lateral hip muscles (the agonist) against resistance.
- After 6 to 10 seconds, the client should relax all muscle groups, which will allow you to further stretch the hip adductors. Hold this stretch for 30 seconds.
- Repeat this technique for 2 to 4 repetitions to maximize muscular flexibility.

Stretching the Piriformis (and the Deep External Rotators of the Hip)

Static Stretching Techniques for the Piriformis

Starting position: The client lies in a supine position with the knees flexed to 90°.

Movement: The client crosses one knee over the top of the other. With both hands, the client grabs behind the knee of the lower leg. The client then pulls the knees toward the chest, holding the stretch for up to 30 seconds.

Dynamic Stretching Techniques for the Piriformis

Trail leg walking (see p. 105)

PNF Stretching Techniques for the Piriformis (and the External and Internal Rotators of the Hip)

The following discussion describes the PNF techniques for the piriformis muscle and the deep external rotators of the hip. PNF for internal rotation of the hip may be performed in the same manner but in the opposite direction.

Hold-Relax (HR)

- Have the client assume a supine position with the legs straight.
- Manually lift one of the client's legs, flexing the hip to 90° and holding the knee at a 90° angle.
- To perform the stretch, maintain the 90-90 hip and knee position while rotating the foot toward the midline. This initial stretch position should be held for up to 10 seconds.
- Ask the client to isometrically contract the hip muscles by attempting to rotate the leg away from the midline. The client holds this position for up to 10 seconds while you apply a matching force in the opposite direction.
- When the client relaxes the contraction, you should immediately passively stretch the muscle beyond the initial stretch position, increasing the stretch on the piriformis. Hold this stretch for 30 seconds.
- Perform 2 to 4 repetitions per muscle or muscle group.

Agonist Contraction

- Have the client assume a supine position with the legs straight.
- Manually lift one of the client's legs, flexing the hip to 90° and holding the knee in a 90° angle.
- To perform the stretch, maintain the 90-90 hip and knee position while rotating the foot toward the midline. Hold the stretch for 10 seconds.
- After the 10-second hold, instruct the client to contract the hip (say "try to rotate your foot toward the midline") while you provide resistance to this movement (place your hands on the medial side of the leg) for 6 to 10 seconds.
- After this isometric contraction, you should again passively rotate the client's hip by rotating the foot toward the midline to stretch the piriformis. Hold the stretch for 30 seconds.
- Perform 2 to 4 agonist contractions per muscle or muscle group.

Hold-Relax With Agonist Contraction

- Have the client assume a supine position with the legs straight.
- Manually lift one of the client's legs, flexing the hip to 90° and holding the knee in a 90° angle.
- To perform the stretch, maintain the 90-90 hip and knee position while rotating the foot toward the midline. This initial stretch position should be held for up to 10 seconds.
- After the client performs the isometric contraction (10 seconds), the client should allow the hip muscles to relax. The client should then immediately actively contract the agonist group against resistance.
- After 6 to 10 seconds, the client should relax all muscle groups, which will allow you to further stretch the piriformis. Hold this stretch for 30 seconds.
- Repeat this technique for 2 to 4 repetitions to maximize muscular flexibility.

Foam Roll Application for the Piriformis

Starting position: The client is sitting as shown, leaning toward the hip that will be stretched. The foot on the same side (same side as the hip to be stretched) is crossed over the opposite knee.

Movement: The client rolls back and forth over the posterior hip region.

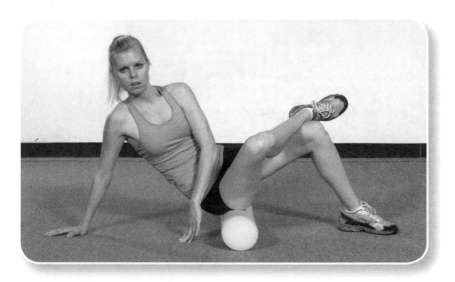

Stretching the Muscles of the Low Back

Static Stretching Techniques for the Muscles of the Low Back

Trunk Rotation

Starting position: The client lies supine with the lower extremities in a hook-lying position (hips flexed to 45° and knees flexed to 90°).

Movement: The client rotates the knees toward the floor, holds the stretch for the desired length of time, and then returns to the starting position. This stretch should be performed to each side.

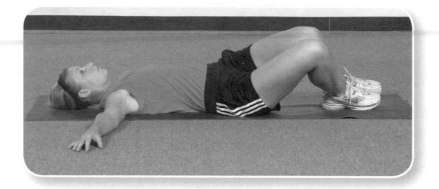

Knee to Chest Stretch

Starting position: The client lies supine in a hook-lying position.

Movement: The client grabs behind the back of both knees, pulling the knees toward the chest. The client should hold the stretch for up to 30 seconds.

Prayer Stretch (and Prayer Stretch With Side Bending)

Starting position: The client starts in the quadruped position.

Movement: The client sits back on the heels with the arms outstretched in front. To emphasize one side of the trunk, the client can maintain the stretching position while walking the hands to the opposite side (opposite from the side to be stretched).

Cobra Pose

Starting position: The client lies in a prone position.

Movement: The client uses his arms to lift his torso off the ground. The abdominal muscles should remain on the surface, and the back muscles should be relaxed. The client holds the position for 30 seconds.

Dynamic Stretching Techniques for the Muscles of the Low Back

Walking lunge (see p. 98)

Walking reverse lunge (see p. 98)

Walking lunge with trunk rotation (see p. 98)

Hand walking (see p. 97)

Foam Roll Application for the Muscles of the Low Back

Starting position: The client lies on top of the foam roll, supporting the upper body with both arms.

Movement: Using the arms and legs, the client rolls along the length of the low back.

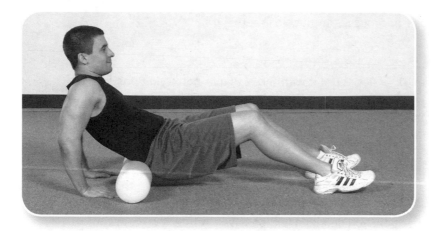

Stretching the Abdominal Muscles

Static Stretching Techniques for the Abdominal Muscles

Starting position 1

Starting position: The client lies in a prone position (this is the same as the cobra pose exercise).

Movement: The client uses the arms to push the torso upward, keeping the hips and pelvis on the floor.

Starting position 2

Starting position: The client lies on the floor in a hook-lying position.

Movement: The client rotates the lower extremities to the side, holding the stretch for 30 seconds. The client should perform this stretch on both sides.

Dynamic Stretching Techniques for the Abdominal Muscles

Walking lunge (see p. 98)

Walking lunge with trunk rotation (see p. 98)

PNF Stretching Techniques for the Abdominal Muscles

Hold-Relax (HR)

- Have the client lie supine on a floor or mat with the legs in a hook-lying position.
- Rotate the client's lower extremities to one side. You should have one hand on the client's shoulder to stabilize the torso. Your other hand should be on the client's knees to guide the torso rotation. To perform the stretch, hold this position. This initial stretch position should be held for up to 10 seconds.

- Ask the client to isometrically contract the abdominal muscles by attempting to rotate her legs toward the center. The client should hold this position for up to 10 seconds while you apply a matching force in the opposite direction.
- When the client relaxes the contraction, you should immediately passively stretch the client's muscles further into the available rotation range. Hold this stretch for 30 seconds.
- Perform 2 to 4 repetitions per muscle or muscle group.

Agonist Contraction

- Have the client lie supine on a floor or mat with the legs in a hook-lying position.
- Rotate the client's lower extremities to one side. You should have one hand on the client's shoulder to stabilize the torso. Your other hand should be on the client's knees to guide the torso rotation. To perform the stretch, hold this position. This initial stretch position should be held for up to 10 seconds.
- After the 10-second hold, instruct the client to contract the abdominal muscles by trying to rotate her legs toward the floor while you provide resistance to this movement (place your hands on the lateral side of the lower leg) for 6 to 10 seconds.
- After this isometric contraction, you should again passively rotate the client toward the floor. Hold the stretch for 30 seconds.
- Perform 2 to 4 agonist contractions per muscle or muscle group.

Hold-Relax With Agonist Contraction

- Have the client lie supine on a floor or mat with the legs in a hook-lying position.
- Rotate the client's lower extremities to one side. You should have one hand on the client's shoulder to stabilize the torso. Your other hand should be on the client's knees to guide the torso rotation. To perform the stretch, hold this position. This initial stretch position should be held for up to 10 seconds.
- After the client performs the isometric contraction (10 seconds), the client should allow the abdominal muscles to relax. The client should then immediately actively contract the agonist group against resistance.
- After 6 to 10 seconds, the client should relax all muscle groups, which will allow you to further stretch the client's abdominal muscles. Hold the stretch for 30 seconds.
- Repeat this technique for 2 to 4 repetitions to maximize muscular flexibility.

Foam Roll Application for the Abdominal Muscles

Because of the proximity of the abdominal organs, using the foam roller over this region is not recommended.

Stretching the Latissimus Dorsi

Static Stretching Technique for the Latissimus Dorsi

Starting position: The client is kneeling on the floor with the arms extended in front of the body (this is the same as the prayer stretch).

Movement: The client sits back on the heels, keeping the torso as close to the floor as possible.

Dynamic Stretching Techniques for the Latissimus Dorsi

Hand walking (see p. 97)

Walking lunge with trunk rotation (see p. 98)

PNF Stretching Techniques for the Latissimus Dorsi

Hold-Relax (HR)

- Have the client assume a sitting position in a chair or on the floor.
- Use one hand to support the client's upper extremity, grasping the upper arm (the shoulder should be maximally flexed with the elbow flexed to 90°). Use the other hand to stabilize the client's torso, placing the hand on the opposite side of the trunk.
- To perform the stretch, gently guide the client's arm behind the head until the client feels a stretch in the latissimus dorsi. This initial stretch position should be held for up to 10 seconds.
- Ask the client to isometrically contract the latissimus dorsi by attempting to pull the arm toward the side of the body. The client should hold this position for up to 10 seconds while you apply a matching force in the opposite direction.
- When the client relaxes the contraction, you should immediately passively stretch the client's arm beyond the initial stretch position, increasing the stretch on the latissimus dorsi. Hold this stretch for 30 seconds.
- Perform 2 to 4 repetitions per muscle or muscle group.

Agonist Contraction

- Have the client assume a sitting position in a chair or on the floor.
- Use one hand to support the client's upper extremity, grasping the upper arm (the shoulder should be completely flexed with the elbow flexed to 90°). Use the other hand to stabilize the client's torso, placing the hand on the opposite side of the trunk.
- To perform the stretch, gently guide the client's arm behind the head until the client feels a stretch in the latissimus dorsi. This initial stretch position should be held for up to 10 seconds.
- After the 10-second hold, instruct the client to move the arm behind the head while you provide resistance to this movement (place your hand to the medial side of the upper arm) for 6 to 10 seconds.
- After this isometric contraction, you should again passively stretch the client's latissimus dorsi. Hold the stretch for 30 seconds.
- Perform 2 to 4 agonist contractions per muscle or muscle group.

Hold-Relax With Agonist Contraction

- Have the client assume a sitting position in a chair or on the floor.
- Use one hand to support the client's upper extremity, grasping the upper arm (the shoulder should be completely flexed with the elbow flexed to 90°). Use the other hand to stabilize the client's torso, placing the hand on the opposite side of the trunk.
- To perform the stretch, gently guide the client's arm behind the head until the client feels a stretch in the latissimus dorsi. This initial stretch position should be held for up to 10 seconds.
- Ask the client to isometrically contract the latissimus dorsi by attempting to pull the arm toward the side of the body. The client should hold this position for up to 10 seconds while you apply a matching force in the opposite direction.
- After the client performs the isometric contraction (10 seconds), the client should allow the latissimus dorsi to relax. The client should then immediately actively contract the agonist group against resistance.
- After 6 to 10 seconds, the client should relax all muscle groups, which will allow you to further stretch the client's latissimus dorsi. Hold the stretch for 30 seconds.
- Repeat this technique for 2 to 4 repetitions to maximize muscular flexibility.

Foam Roll Application for the Latissimus Dorsi

The following foam roll application addresses the latissimus dorsi and the upper back region in general.

Starting position: The client is positioned with the upper back resting on the foam roll. The hips should be flexed to approximately 45°, the knees bent to approximately 90°, and the feet resting on the floor.

Movement: Using the legs and contralateral arm, the client rolls from the upper back (axilla) to the middle back.

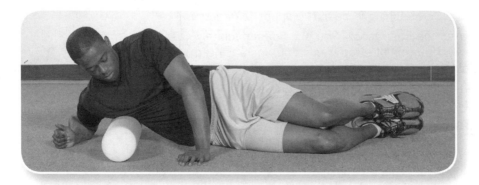

SUMMARY

Optimal flexibility is essential for all clients, athletes, and patients. Improved core flexibility will help manual laborers use proper lifting postures. Correcting flexibility deficits can help athletes improve their sport performance. And, increasing range of motion will help patients recover from orthopedic surgery.

However, many clients fail to incorporate flexibility exercises into their training program. Those who do stretch will often stretch infrequently or perform the techniques incorrectly. The role of the fitness professional is to identify potential deficits and then apply the optimal mode of stretching to maximize the client's flexibility. The fitness professional must also stay abreast of the latest flexibility trends and fads, comparing these new approaches with evidence-supported techniques and the scientific advances reported in the research literature.

8

Plyometric Training

The inclusion of plyometric exercises in an athlete's training program is crucial for improving performance in sports. These exercises, when performed correctly, are designed to develop explosive power in athletes.

HISTORY OF PLYOMETRICS

During the 1960s and 1970s, athletes from Eastern European countries and the Soviet Union dominated Olympic sports such as track and field, weightlifting, and gymnastics (Chu 1998; Chu and Cordier 2000). The Eastern Europeans and the Soviets were using a new form of exercise that helped to provide a competitive edge in sports that require speed and power. This new form of exercise was called *shock method* or *jump training*. Jump training (now known as plyometrics) can be attributed to then Soviet Union coach and researcher Yuri Verkhoshansky. His early publications on jump training introduced the rest of the world to the benefits of plyometrics.

Fred Wilt, an American track coach, changed the name of jump training to plyometrics (Chu and Cordier 2000). Chu describes plyometrics as the exercise form that "enables a muscle to reach maximum strength in as short a time as possible" (Chu 1998, p. 2). This has obvious implications for sports. For example, a basketball forward who can jump high *and* quickly will likely be able to outrebound his opponent. Because of its role in linking strength with speed of movement, plyometric training must be included in any athlete's periodized training program (Radcliffe and Farentinos 1999; Potach and Chu 2000).

THE SCIENCE BEHIND PLYOMETRICS

Researchers have proposed two models to explain how plyometrics enhances power development in athletes (Potach and Chu 2000). In the **mechanical model,** elastic energy (form of energy created when a structure is stretched [e.g.. muscle and tendon unit]) is stored and subsequently released from the **series elastic component (SEC).** The SEC consists of the tendon and the associated connective tissue. In the **neurophysiological model,** stimulation of muscle spindles initiates a reflex response that ultimately contributes to an increase in force production. The **muscle spindle,** a proprioceptive organ, responds to changes in the rate and magnitude of a stretch applied to a muscle. This reflex increases the activity of the muscle that was stretched, consequently increasing the force produced.

Both the mechanical and neurophysiological models are believed to be simultaneously contributing to force production, but the percentage of contribution from each model is unknown (Potach and Chu 2000).

Plyometric exercises, then, involve a "quick, powerful movement using a prestretch, or countermovement, that involves the stretch-shortening cycle" (Potach and Chu 2000, p. 414). Correctly using the stretch-shortening cycle, one of the fastest reflexes in the human body, is key to maximizing the training effects from plyometrics. The three phases of the stretch-shortening cycle are the eccentric phase, the amortization phase, and the concentric phase. Within each phase, aspects of both the mechanical and neurophysiological models are at play. Let's take a closer look at the physiological aspects of each phase.

The first phase, the eccentric phase, occurs when the agonist muscle group is preloaded. An eccentric contraction is performed, applying a stretch to the SEC. At this point, the muscle spindles have been stimulated, and the SEC is lengthened, storing elastic energy (Potach and Chu 2000). The second phase is the amortization phase, which represents the period of time between the eccentric and concentric phases. Although researchers do not specify exactly how long the amortization phase should last, there is consensus that it must be as short as possible (Chu 1998). Wasting time transitioning from the eccentric phase to the concentric phase will prevent the athlete from taking advantage of the stretch reflex and will waste stored energy. In the final phase, the concentric phase, the athlete uses the energy released from the SEC and the **potentiation** from the stretch reflex to maximize the force output.

A sample plyometric exercise (the depth jump) can be used to demonstrate the role of the quadriceps muscle during each phase of the stretch-shortening cycle. The athlete, initially standing on top of a box, steps off the box and lands with both feet on the floor. The athlete's landing position creates an eccentric (or lengthening) contraction of the quadriceps muscle. After the landing, the athlete must immediately perform a vertical jump. The jumping component of this plyometric exercise creates a concentric (or shortening) contraction of the quadriceps. The crucial period of time between the eccentric and concentric phases of this exercise is the amortization phase. (Note: Although this example focuses specifically on the role of the quadriceps muscle, you should not forget that muscles throughout the lower kinetic chain contribute to this function.)

Research Evidence Supporting the Prescription of Plyometric Training

A study was conducted to determine the effects of a physical conditioning program on club head speed in NCAA Division I golfers. Sixteen golfers (10 men and 6 women) participated in a supervised training program for strength, power, and flexibility (Doan et al. 2006). The golfers exercised three times a week for 11 weeks. The training program included two plyometric exercises for the trunk: medicine ball speed rotations and medicine ball standing throws. The golfers also performed a trunk strengthening program during each session. Significant pretest-to-posttest increases were noted in each of the strength, power, and flexibility tests. Club head speed improved significantly, increasing driving distance approximately 4.9 meters (16 feet). The researchers concluded that the program (consisting of flexibility training, strength training, and plyometric exercises) significantly increased a golfer's club head speed without affecting putting distance control in collegiate golfers.

Other researchers studied the effects of a weight training and plyometric program on golf performance (Fletcher and Hartwell 2004). Six male golfers participated in an 8-week training program. The participants' club head speed and driving distance were tested before and after the 8-week training program. The strengthening program consisted of the following exercises for the trunk: abdominal crunches, back extension, and side bends. Four medicine ball exercises were also performed: seated and standing horizontal twists, standing back extensions, and golf swings. Controls showed no significant changes, whereas the training group demonstrated a significant increase ($p \leq 0.05$) in club head speed and driving distance. The researchers thought that the changes in driving performance resulted from an increase in muscular force and an improvement in the sequential acceleration of body parts contributing to a greater final velocity being applied to the ball. The researchers concluded that a weight training and plyometric program can help increase club head speed and driving distance in golfers.

PRINCIPLES OF PLYOMETRIC PROGRAM DESIGN

When designing a plyometric training program, you must consider each of the following variables:

- **Mode.** Mode refers to the region of the body to be trained. Modes are defined as lower body, upper body, and trunk.

- **Intensity.** Intensity is based on the forces applied to the joint and is usually described as low, medium, or high.

- **Frequency.** Frequency refers to the number of training sessions performed each week. Although standard practice is to have athletes perform plyometric exercises one to three times a week, research has yet to determine how many sessions are the most effective.

- **Recovery.** Recovery relates to the amount of time an athlete should rest between reps, sets, and workouts. The recommended work-to-rest ratio is 1:5 or 1:10. If an exercise requires 10 seconds to complete, the athlete should rest 50 to 100 seconds between sets (Chu and Cordier 2000). Athletes should rest 1 to 5 minutes between each different exercise (Stone and O'Bryant 1987; Potach and Chu 2000). The accepted rest period between sessions is 48 to 72 hours. Plyometric exercises for the same body region should not be done on back-to-back days.

- **Volume.** Volume relates to the number of repetitions and sets to be performed at any particular training session. Beginners often perform fewer sets and reps than advanced athletes. The number of repetitions and sets you prescribe will also be dependent on the training phase (e.g., off-season, preseason, and so on). For example, a beginner may perform 60 to 100 repetitions (foot contacts) of low- to moderate-intensity exercises for the lower extremities during the hypertrophy–endurance phase of the preparatory period (Chu 1998).

Unfortunately, little research is available regarding the most effective training volume for trunk-specific plyometric exercises. Many plyometric exercises for the trunk involve throwing and catching a medicine ball. Some researchers suggest establishing a training volume based on the number of throws performed with each upper extremity drill (Potach and Chu 2000). Many of the trunk exercises use upper extremity throws. When initiating a trunk-specific plyometric program for an athlete, you should consider initially prescribing 2 or 3 sets of 10 repetitions. If the athlete is able to recover without excessive muscle soreness, you can advance the number of reps and sets as necessary.

- **Program length.** The ideal program length for a plyometric training program has not been definitively identified. Researchers have suggested that anywhere from 4 to 10 weeks of training is required to maximize outcomes (Potach and Chu 2000).

- **Progression.** Progression refers to progressively overloading a muscle or muscle group. For example, you may start an athlete at a low to moderate volume of exercises at low intensity. You can later progress the athlete toward high-intensity exercises to mimic the demands of his sport.

PREREQUISITES TO PLYOMETRIC TRAINING

Before initiating a plyometric training program, the client or athlete should have some level of functional strength (Potach and Chu 2000). For example, some reports suggest that a client must be able to perform a 1-repetition max (1RM) squat at a minimum weight of one and a half times his body weight before being allowed to begin lower body plyometric training (Holcomb et al. 1998; National Strength and Conditioning Association 1993; Wathen 1993). Based on this criteria, a 200-pound individual must be able to squat at least 300 pounds before being allowed to perform a high-intensity plyometric exercise for the lower body. However, this guideline appears to be based only on clinical commentary reports, not on research evidence. Clinical commentary reports are published expert opinions. These reports serve a role in the dissemination of knowledge but are limited by the fact that they have not been challenged by the research process. Potach and Chu (2000, p. 424) report that for athletes "who (do) not possess sufficient muscular strength or a sufficient fitness level, plyometrics should be delayed until they meet minimum standards." Unfortunately, this fails to address when someone should be allowed to begin a plyometric program. The recommendations put forth by Allerheiligen and Rogers (1995) could help to guide clinical decision making (see the guidelines below). In addition, recent research reports have described the use of low-, medium-, and high-intensity plyometrics focused on the lower extremities. In these reports, the exercise program was progressed over a 6-week period as part of an injury prevention program. The results indicate that this training was applied successfully to a variety of trained and untrained athletes without negative side effects (Hewett et al. 1996; Hewett et al. 1999).

OTHER TRAINING CONSIDERATIONS

Some people suggest that plyometric exercises should not be performed by children. These people believe that plyometric training may damage a child's joints. However, little research has been done to investigate injury risk with plyometric training. Are children really at risk for injury? What do kids do all day? They jump, they skip, they hop, and they throw. Although the risk of injury is probably low, Allerheiligen and Rogers (1995) developed a classification system that helps to guide the strength training professional when prescribing plyometrics to the adolescent athlete. This same classification system may also be utilized when prescribing plyometrics for rehab patients, general clients, and athletes. The system includes three categories:

■ **Beginners:** A beginner has no previous experience performing plyometrics. A person is classified as a beginner if she is unskilled, has not reached puberty, or is a rehab client. These clients should begin with low-intensity plyometric exercises.

■ **Intermediate:** The intermediate classification includes people of high school age as well as patients who are in the later stages of their rehabilitation progression (e.g., someone who is no longer experiencing joint or muscle pain and has been cleared by a physician to resume all normal activity). These individuals may perform medium-intensity plyometric exercises or drills.

■ **Advanced:** The advanced classification includes collegiate and elite athletes. These athletes may perform high-intensity plyometrics. High-intensity plyometrics are not suggested for rehabilitation clients.

The National Strength and Conditioning Association (NSCA) has also developed a position statement that provides further guidance for when to implement plyometric training programs. This position statement can be found at http://www.nsca-lift.org/Publications/posstatements.shtml.

Following is the position of the National Strength and Conditioning Association:

1. The stretch-shortening cycle, characterized by a rapid deceleration of a mass followed almost immediately by rapid acceleration of the mass in the opposite direction, is essential in the performance of most competitive sports, particularly those involving running, jumping, and rapid changes in direction.

2. A plyometric exercise program that trains the muscles, connective tissue, and nervous system to effectively carry out the stretch-shortening cycle can improve performance in most competitive sports.

3. A plyometric training program for athletes should include sport-specific exercises.

4. Carefully applied plyometric exercise programs are no more harmful than other forms of sport training and competition, and they may be necessary for safe adaptation to the rigors of explosive sports.

5. Only athletes who have already achieved high levels of strength through standard resistance training should engage in plyometric drills.

6. Depth jumps should only be used by a small percentage of athletes engaged in plyometric training. As a rule, athletes weighing over 220 pounds should not depth jump from platforms higher than 18 inches.

7. Plyometric drills involving a particular muscle or joint complex should not be performed on consecutive days.

8. Plyometric drills should not be performed when an athlete is fatigued. Time for complete recovery should be allowed between plyometric exercise sets.

9. Footwear and landing surfaces used in plyometric drills must have good shock-absorbing qualities.

10. A thorough set of warm-up exercises should be performed before beginning a plyometric training session. Less demanding drills should be mastered prior to attempting more complex and intense drills.

Reprinted, by permission, from NSCA. Available: http://www.nsca-lift.org/Publications/posstatements.shtml

PLYOMETRIC EXERCISES

Plyometric exercises or drills should be included in the training program for all athletes (see table 8.1). Even though plyometric drills are often classified by the body region exercised (i.e., lower body, upper body, or trunk), many exercises that are classified as "lower body" or "upper body" also train the core. For example, the side throw (an upper body drill) would be an appropriate exercise to include in a golfer's plyometric training program.

Many of the exercises presented in this section require the use of a medicine ball and possibly either a **rebounder** or a partner. Instruct your client or athlete to perform an abdominal brace before each set of repetitions.

Table 8.1 Plyometric Exercises, Intensity Level, and Indications for Sport

Exercise	Intensity	Sport
Underhand throw	Low	Football, wrestling
Overhead throw	Low	Baseball, track (throwing events)
Trunk rotation	Low	All sports
Side throw	Low	All sports
Backward throw	Low	Wrestling, track (throwing events)
Medicine ball twists	Low	Football, wrestling, throwing sports
Medicine ball over and under	Low	Wrestling
Medicine ball seated side throws	Low	All sports
Medicine ball reach-ups	Low	All sports
Pull-over pass	Medium	Throwing sports
Medicine ball sit-up	Medium	All sports
Twist and touch	Medium.	All sports
Sit-up and throw	Medium	All sports
Vertical swing	High	Sports with jumps
Medicine ball scoop toss	High	All sports

Underhand Throw

Starting position: Client is squatting, holding the medicine ball slightly in front of the body and close to the ground

Movement: The client quickly stands (explodes) up from the squatting position, using the power generated from the legs to help perform the underhand throw.

Common errors: Some clients may be unable to maintain a neutral spine posture throughout the motion. You should stand approximately 9 to 12 feet (2.7 to 3.6 m) away in order to observe the client's posture during this exercise.

Intensity: Low

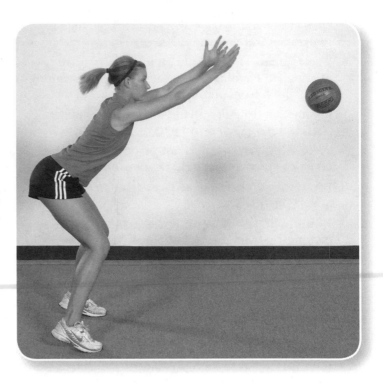

Overhead Throw

Starting position: Standing, facing either a rebounder or a partner, and holding a medicine ball overhead

Movement: The client steps forward and passes the medicine ball to the partner or at the rebounder.

Intensity: Low

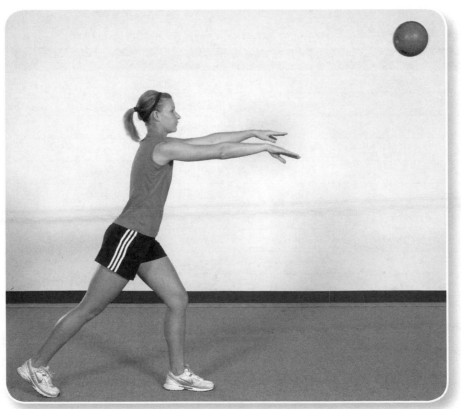

Trunk Rotation

Starting position: Client is sitting with her legs abducted as far from the midline as possible. A partner holds a medicine ball behind the client's back.

Movement: The client rotates to the ball, grabs it, and then rotates the ball to the opposite side, handing the ball to the partner. This should be performed to each side for the desired number of repetitions.

Intensity: Low

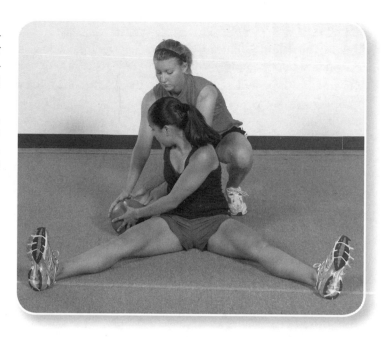

Side Throw

Starting position: Standing in a ready position and holding the medicine ball with both hands

Movement: The client initiates the movement by rotating the ball away from the target (partner or rebounder). The client then rapidly changes directions, rotating back toward the partner or rebounder and throwing the ball.

Variation: The client may perform the side throw while in a kneeling position.

Intensity: Low

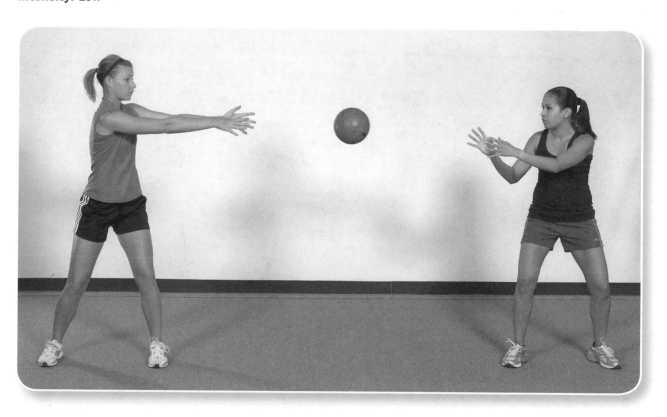

Backward Throw

Starting position: Squatting while holding the medicine ball between the legs. A partner is standing approximately 9 to 12 feet (2.7 to 3.6 m) behind the athlete.

Movement: The client stands up and throws the ball back over his head to the partner.

Common errors: A client may round (excessively flex) the back while squatting, instead of maintaining a neutral spine.

Intensity: Low

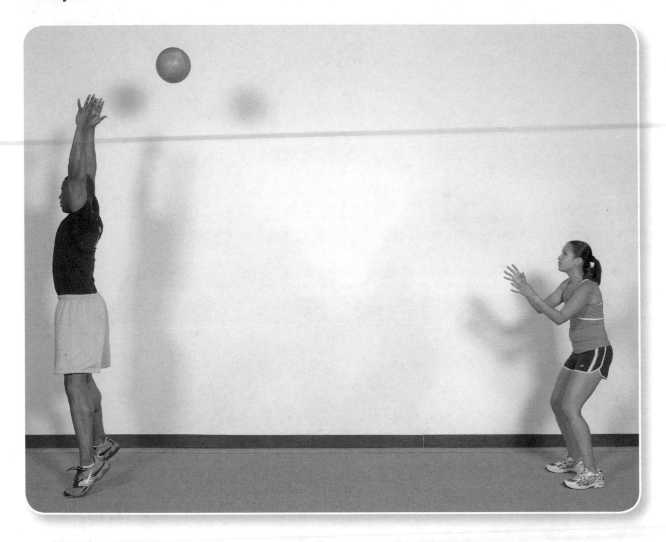

Medicine Ball Twists

Starting position: Standing back to back with a partner while holding the medicine ball

Movement: The client rotates in order to hand the medicine ball to one side for the partner to grab. This is repeated to each side for the desired number of repetitions.

Intensity: Low

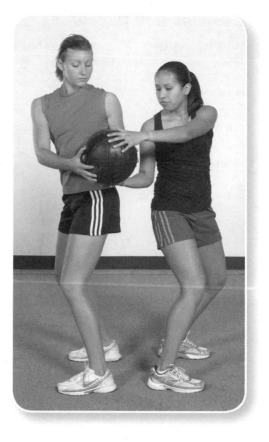

Medicine Ball Seated Side Throw

Starting position: Seated and facing the same or opposite direction from a partner who is approximately 5 to 6 feet (152 to 183 cm) away. The client is holding a medicine ball with both hands.

Movement: The client rotates his torso to the side opposite the partner, touches the floor with the ball, then quickly rotates toward the partner and throws the ball. After catching the ball, the partner repeats the same sequence.

Intensity: Low

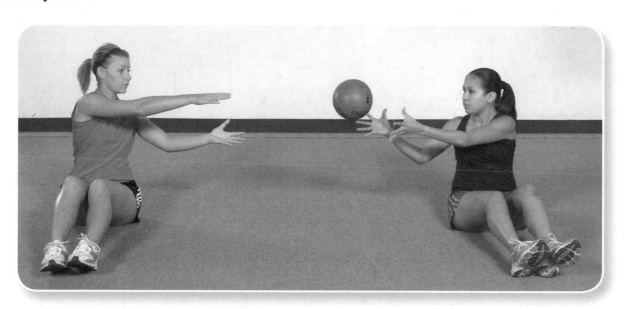

Medicine Ball Reach-Ups

Starting position: Lying supine with the hips and knees bent. A partner stands to one side of the athlete (near the athlete's waistline). The partner is holding a medicine ball.

Movement: The client performs a partial sit-up, reaching for the ball. The client grabs the ball and returns to the starting position. The partner then reaches down to take the ball from the client.

Intensity: Low

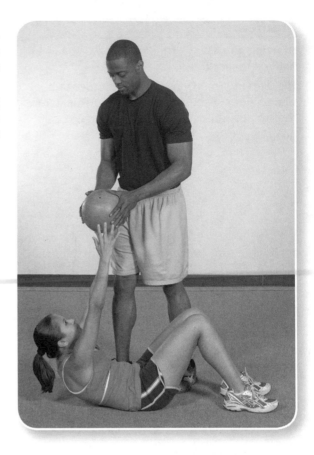

Pull-Over Pass

Starting position: Lying supine with the knees bent. The client is holding a medicine ball with both arms extended overhead. A partner stands at the client's feet.

Movement: The client rises up and throws (passes) the ball to the partner while keeping the arms extended.

Intensity: Medium

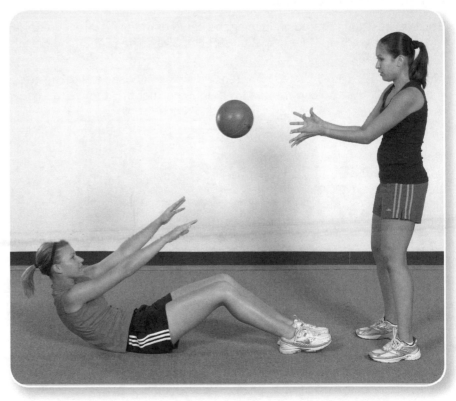

Medicine Ball Sit-Up

Starting position: Sitting approximately 3 to 4 feet (91 to 122 cm) away from a partner. The client and the partner are facing each other, and both have their knees flexed. The client begins in a supine position, holding the medicine ball.

Movement: The client starts by performing a sit-up, rising from the supine position and throwing the ball to the partner. The partner catches the ball near the top of the sit-up position. The partner allows the ball's momentum to lower him to the ground, then quickly reverses direction, performs a sit-up, and throws the ball back to the client.

Intensity: Medium

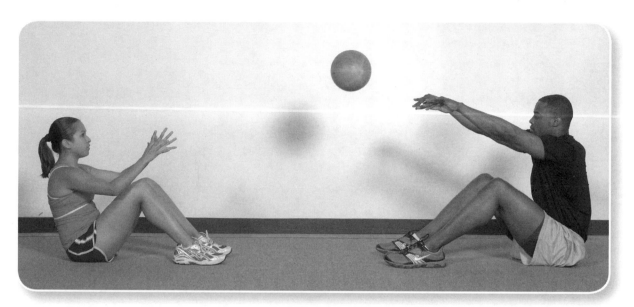

Twist and Touch

Starting position: Sitting in a V position with the feet off the ground. The partner stands behind and to the side of the client.

Movement: The client begins by holding the medicine ball on the ground (near his hip) on the side opposite the partner. The client rotates the ball across his body toward the partner, touching the partner's hand, then returns the ball back to the starting position. The client repeats this movement to both sides for the desired number of repetitions.

Intensity: Medium

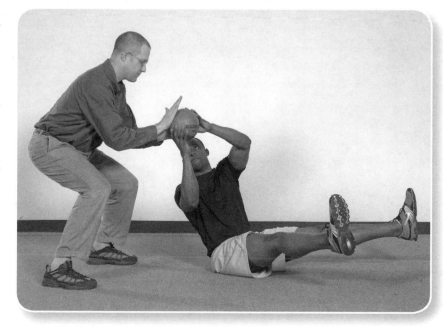

Sit-Up and Throw

Starting position: Sitting on the floor with the hips and knees bent. A partner stands approximately 2 to 3 feet (61 to 91 cm) away, holding a medicine ball.

Movement: The partner throws the ball to the client's hands, while the client lowers his body toward the floor. The client catches the ball and completes his descent to the floor. Once on the floor, the client reverses the maneuver, sitting up and throwing the ball back to the partner.

Intensity: Medium

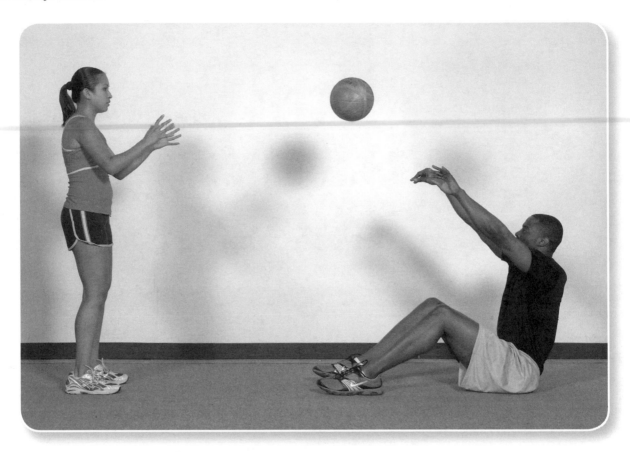

Vertical Swing

Starting position: The client assumes a standing position, holding a kettleball or medicine ball with both hands.

Movement: The client lifts the kettleball or medicine ball with outstretched arms over her head, then reverses the direction pulling the kettleball downward while the body assumes a deep squat position. She then explodes out of this position, lifting the kettleball overhead. Repeat this sequence for the desired number of repetitions.

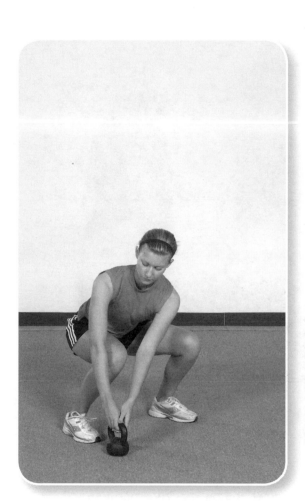

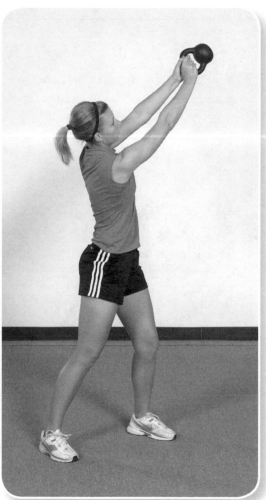

Medicine Ball Scoop Toss

Starting position: Client stands with feet hip-width apart in an athletic ready-position (knees bent approximately 20° to 30°). A partner stands beside the client, 4 to 5 feet away and facing the same direction.

Movement: The client starts with the medicine ball on one side at hip level, then tosses the ball to a partner allowing the upper body to rotate only slightly. The partner will catch the ball and repeat the same sequence, throwing the ball back. Repeat to both sides of the body for the desired number of repetitions.

Intensity: High

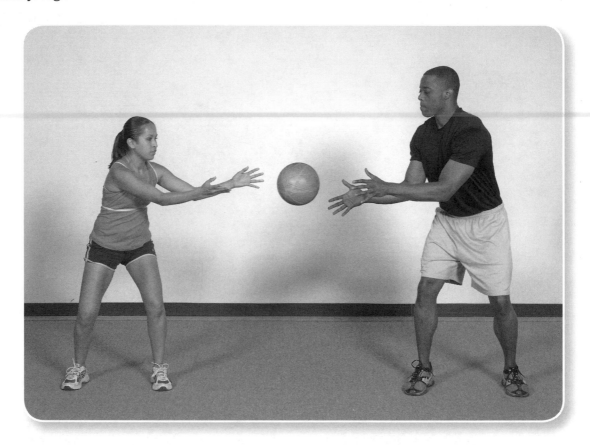

SUMMARY

The difference between a win and a loss may come down to how quickly an athlete can get a ball, how far he can jump, or how far he can hit a ball. Plyometric exercises are key to developing the explosive power required to improve sport performance. Recent research has highlighted the functional benefits of including plyometrics for the core in the athlete's training program.

These exercises should be included as a part of every athlete's training program. Before initiating a plyometric training program, you must give careful consideration to the athlete's experience level. With proper manipulation of the plyometric training variables, most athletes will be able to safely perform these valuable exercises.

9

Special Considerations for Core Training

The muscles and joints of the core are frequently injured in both athletic and nonathletic individuals. Millions of dollars are spent each year on medical and therapeutic treatments to help return injured individuals back to full function. In some cases an injury may be so severe that restoration of normal function is not possible.

The purpose of this chapter is to present common musculoskeletal injuries to the core region. The exercise programs you develop for postrehab clients will be influenced by their recent and previous medical history. In addition, this chapter will address core training issues related to pregnancy and to specific athletic populations.

INJURIES TO THE CORE AND TRAINING CONSIDERATIONS

Musculoskeletal injuries to the core account for a significant portion of all injuries treated by physicians and rehabilitation professionals. Low back pain (LBP), in particular, will affect up to 80% of Americans at least once in their lifetime (Rasmussen-Barr et al. 2003). Many injuries to the core are successfully rehabilitated with conservative treatments; however, some injuries may require significant recovery periods. In certain cases, surgical interventions may be necessary for an individual to return to normal function. Exercise programs implemented by a fitness professional may help facilitate a **postrehab** client's return to work or sport and may help to reduce a client's risk of reinjury.

Being familiar with common back and hip injuries will improve how you design core training programs for your clients. As always, you should review each client's medical history (especially any history of musculoskeletal injury or pain)

before initiating a training program. If the client has a musculoskeletal injury, refer the client to an appropriate medical provider. If therapy is necessary, it is the role of the rehabilitation professional to treat specific injuries. Some patients who have been discharged from therapy may not be at an optimal functional level. A patient may be prematurely discharged from therapy for a host of reasons. It is the fitness professional who will have the opportunity to develop and implement a postrehab training program for the asymptomatic client who has had recent or incompletely rehabilitated musculoskeletal injury.

The following sections provide information about common injuries experienced in the back and hips. For each injury, a brief explanation of the pathomechanics is provided, along with suggestions for prevention or postrehab training. Despite the suggested tips, remember that you must still interview the client and perform a functional assessment.

Spine Injuries

The following sections provide detail about some of the more common musculoskeletal injuries to the spine. Significant pain and disability may result from some of these injuries. The fitness professional who develops a core training program for a client with a history of back pain must address the client's potential strength limitations while avoiding the prescription of exercises that may reaggravate the condition.

Lumbar muscle strain

A strain involves an overstretching or tearing of muscle tissue. Muscle strains are usually caused by excessive tension or stress applied to the muscle beyond what it can sustain (figure 9.1).

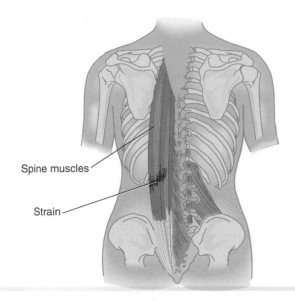

Spine muscles

Strain

Figure 9.1 A lumbar muscle strain.

Reprinted, by permission, from M. Flegel, 2008, *Sport first aid,* 4th ed. (Champaign, IL: Human Kinetics), 191.

For example, repeatedly lifting a heavy object with incorrect technique or using faulty postures (such as excessive lumbar lordosis) can contribute to lumbar muscle strains. Clients or athletes who have sustained a strain in the thoracic or lumbar spine may experience pain and stiffness that can impair their functional ability. This often leads individuals to seek treatment from a rehabilitation specialist. Be sure to ask whether a client has recently participated in a rehabilitation program. If this is the case, you should also find out what exercises the client learned from the rehabilitation specialist.

Common dysfunctional patterns and typical assessment findings:

- Pain with flexion and side bending movements
- Pain or an inability to lift objects off of the ground
- Muscle guarding or spasming in the low back
- Pain with palpation to the low back muscles

Core training indications

After a strain injury, the client may have residual muscle weakness and may be less flexible in the lumbar region. These limitations should be addressed initially with static stretching and basic core stabilization exercises.

- Static stretching
  - Knee to chest stretch
  - Prayer stretch and prayer stretch with side bending
  - Cobra pose
- Basic core stabilization exercises
  - Bridging
  - Straight-arm pull-downs
  - Side bridge (beginner)
  - Crunch

Core training contraindications

Avoid prescribing exercises that reproduce a client's pain symptoms. Gradually progress the client from basic stabilization exercises to the intermediate level.

Herniated nucleus pulposus (herniated disc)

A herniated nucleus pulposus (HNP) can be a severely debilitating condition, possibly requiring surgery to alleviate symptoms. A disc herniation may range in severity from a **disc protrusion** to a **disc sequestration** (table 9.1).

How do disc injuries occur? Think of the intervertebral disc as a jelly doughnut. The inner jelly portion is the gelatinous nucleus pulposus, and the doughnut portion (the outer border of the disc) is the annulus fibrosus.

What happens to a jelly doughnut when you damage the outer pastry portion? The jelly tends to migrate or spill out. Although this is an oversimplification, a similar process occurs in disc-related

Table 9.1 Types of Disc Injuries

Disc injury	Definition
Disc protrusion	The inner portion of the disc bulges toward the periphery pushing against the outer portion of the disc without disruption of the disc.
Disc extrusion	The outer part of the disc breaks down with disruption of the inner disc.
Disc sequestration	The inner portion of the disc is disrupted and becomes separated from the disc.

injuries. Repetitive stress, such as poor lifting mechanics at work or in the gym, may contribute to the degeneration of the annulus fibrosus (outer doughnut). This can lead to a disc bulge (protrusion of the jelly, see figure 2.4, p. 12), or in a worst-case scenario, the inner portion of the disc can be disrupted and become separated from the disc (disc sequestration).

Common dysfunctional patterns and typical assessment findings

- Pain in the low back, possibly radiating into the leg
- Pain with flexion and side bending motions
- Muscle spasms and guarding in the low back and the gluteal muscles

Core training indications

Most clients with a diagnosis of a lumbar disc injury have previously received treatment from a rehabilitation professional. Despite a course of therapy, clients may continue to experience intermittent pain, a lack of flexibility in the low back or lower extremities, and dysfunctional core strength. Initially, avoid flexion-based exercises such as the crunch. Gradually introduce flexion-based exercises as needed for the client's function. Do not continue an exercise if the client experiences pain.

- Stretching (initial)
  - Cobra pose
  - Supine hamstring stretch
  - Cat and camel
- Basic core stabilization exercises
  - Bird dog
  - Side bridge (beginners)
  - Front plank

Core training contraindications

A client with a herniated lumbar disc may need to avoid certain training exercises. Specifically, the client may need to avoid exercises that could increase the risk of reherniation if performed incorrectly or while unsupervised (Ostelo et al. 2003).

Follow these guidelines for prescribing trunk flexion exercises (abdominal crunches):

- These exercises should be avoided if the client is experiencing acute disc-related pain.

- To address a weak rectus abdominis, initially choose exercises such as the front plank that avoid flexion through the spine
- Hip strengthening is crucial for clients with a history of a herniated disc. Optimal hip strength is necessary to allow an individual to perform a functional squat for sport or work in order to avoid flexion-based movements in the lumbar spine.
- Once the client is pain free, flexion exercises should be used on a case-by-case basis and with caution.

Spondylolysis or spondylolisthesis

Spondylolysis is a defect in the **pars interarticularis**. Spondylolysis can occur bilaterally. In these cases, the vertebra loses the ability to provide posterior stability (figure 9.2a). The result may be slipping of one vertebra anterior to the distal segment. When this slipping occurs, it is called spondylolisthesis (figure 9.2b).

Common dysfunctional patterns and typical assessment findings

- Pain in the low back
- Pain with lumbar extension
- Poor core endurance capacity

Core training indications

A client may be able to perform stretching and strengthening exercises in flexed and neutral spine postures. Extension of the lumbar spine should be avoided. The following are examples of potentially appropriate exercises for a client with spondylolysis or spondylolisthesis:

- Stretching
  - Knee to chest
  - Prayer stretch and prayer stretch with side bending
  - Supine hamstring stretches
  - Piriformis
- Strengthening
  - Bird dog
  - Side bridge (intermediate)
  - Crunch

Core training contraindications

For clients with a history of spondylolisthesis, exercises that extend the spine beyond neutral postures should be avoided.

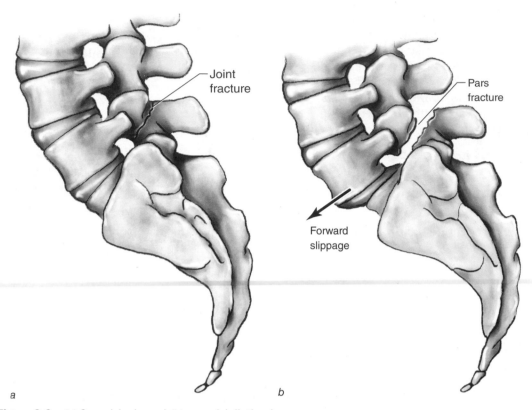

Figure 9.2 *(a)* Spondylosis and *(b)* spondylolisthesis.

Reprinted, by permission, from R. Gotlin, 2008, *Sport injuries guidebook* (Champaign, IL: Human Kinetics), 160, 188.

Hip Injuries

Athletic and sedentary individuals are at risk for hip injuries. Even minor muscle strains can cause pain and impair one's gait and function. Residual hip weakness can alter lower extremity biomechanics, possibly contributing to knee or foot pain. The following sections provide details about some of the more common musculoskeletal injuries to the hip.

Muscle strains of the hip

Hip muscle strains are frequently experienced by competitive and recreational athletes (Tyler et al. 2001; Tyler et al. 2002; Anderson et al. 2001; Grote et al. 2004). Training programs that address pre-season functional limitations may help to reduce the risk of these injuries (Tyler et al. 2002). Table 9.2 presents the injury mechanisms of common hip muscle strains; this table also identifies the

Table 9.2 Common Hip Muscle Strains and the Injury Mechanisms

Muscle or muscle group	Mechanism of injury	Sport
Hip flexors	1. Flexing the hip against a force or a violent hyperextension 2. Violent hit to the anterior hip	• Soccer kick • Football
Hip adductors	1. Quick or strong abduction of the hip during ice skating, hockey, or soccer	• Breaststroke kick • Ice hockey • Ice skating • Cross-country skiing • Football • Soccer
Rectus femoris	1. Flexing the hip against a force 2. Violent or sudden hyperextension	• Soccer kick • Sprinting

Anderson et al. 2001; Tyler et al. 2001; Grote et al. 2004.

sports in which athletes often experience these strains.

The same forces and mechanisms that cause a muscle strain can cause an avulsion (a separation of the muscle from the bone) of the muscle in children and adolescents (Anderson et al. 2001). Children, adolescents, and young teenagers who complain of a "muscle injury" should be referred to a physician to rule out an avulsion injury.

Hip Flexor Strain

A hip flexor (iliacus and psoas major muscles) strain results from a hip flexion movement against a force or a violent hyperextension (Anderson et al. 2001). In addition, a violent hit to the anterior hip (e.g. football tackle) may also cause a hip flexor injury.

Common dysfunctional patterns and typical assessment findings

- Pain in the front of the hip
- Pain with hip flexion
- Pain and a lack of flexibility as the hip is extended
- Loss of hip flexion strength

Core training indications

Hip flexor muscle strains will require both flexibility and strengthening exercises in order to restore function.

- Stretching
- Kneeling hip flexor stretch
- Strengthening
- Standing hip flexion (resistance provided by ankle weights or a machine)
- Lunges
- Side bridge with hip flexion

Hip Adductor Strains

Hip adductor strains are common in sports played on ice or snow and with swimmers who perform the breaststroke (Tyler et al. 2001; Tyler et al. 2002; Grote et al. 2004). Quick or strong abduction of the hip during a sport movement may cause a hip adductor strain.

Common dysfunctional patterns and typical assessment findings

- Pain in the groin region
- Pain with active hip adduction and passive hip abduction

Core training indications

Prevention is the best medicine, but if a strain has occurred, a gentle, gradual stretching program combined with functional strengthening will help return the athlete to sport participation.

- Stretching
  - Sitting groin stretch
  - Side lunge stretch
- Strengthening
  - Squats
  - Side lunges
  - Chu's lunge series for athletes

Rectus Femoris Strain

A strain of the rectus femoris has a similar mechanism to the hip flexor strain. Flexing the hip against a force or violent or sudden hyperextension can injure this muscle. This is one of the primary strains experienced by sprinters.

Common dysfunctional patterns and typical assessment findings

- Pain in the front of the hip and thigh
- Pain with active hip flexion and knee extension
- Pain with passive hip extension
- Loss of motion into hip extension

Core training indications

Individuals who have had a hip flexor strain may benefit from this set of exercises.

- Stretching
  - Standing quadricep stretch
  - Kneeling hip flexor stretch
- Strengthening
  - Squats
  - Lunges

Core training contraindications

If the client is experiencing residual symptoms, avoid exercises that excessively extend the hip and heavy hip flexion and knee extension strengthening exercises.

Hernias

Although hernias are not a musculoskeletal injury, a hernia may be initially mistaken as a muscular strain. If an athlete experiences pain in the groin region during exercise and has not experienced a trauma, this athlete may be suffering from athletic pubalgia, or a sports hernia.

Common dysfunctional patterns and typical assessment findings

- Pain in the groin region
- Pain with coughing or sneezing
- Pain with exercise

Core training indications

Clients may present as if they experienced a hip adductor strain. At some point in the training progression exercise will become painful. A referral to a primary care provider will be necessary to diagnose a hernia.

Core training contraindications

When a client experiences pain with exercise, refer him to the appropriate medical provider (M.D., D.O., N.P., P.A.)

Snapping Hip Syndrome

Snapping hip syndrome received its name because of the "snapping" sound heard from the hip as the iliotibial band pathologically rubs over the greater trochanter during hip flexion and extension (Anderson et al. 2001). This condition primarily affects runners.

Core training indications

Athletes who have this condition (or have had it in the past) will benefit from stretching the ITB and strengthening the hip abductors.

- Stretching
  - Standing ITB stretch
  - Foam roll application for the ITB
- Strengthening
  - Side-lying hip abduction
  - Side planks (intermediate)

Core training contraindications

Progress the client as tolerated. Avoid exercises that reproduce symptoms.

Osteoarthritis of the Hip

A normal consequence of aging is the degenerative changes that occur in the joints. The degenerative changes at a joint may include a loss of the cartilage that cushions the joint, the development of bony spurs, and the occurrence of bone-on-bone contact during weight bearing. Clients who complain of hip pain with the pain worsening through the

day may be experiencing hip osteoarthritis (OA). Hip OA usually does not affect younger people. The earliest onset of symptoms occurs in the fourth decade of life. Clients who have OA should consult an orthopedic surgeon. Several conservative measures may be taken that can help reduce a client's pain. Pain-free core training and general fitness improvements may be helpful. For many, a hip replacement surgery may be necessary.

Common dysfunctional patterns and typical assessment findings

- Pain in the hip
- Pain with walking
- Pain with functional activities
- Loss of range of motion

Core training indications

Strengthening the muscles of the hip may help to reduce pain. However, depending upon the severity of the OA, you may be limited to training the patient in nonweightbearing postures.

Core training contraindications

Avoid exercises that reproduce pain.

THE CORE AND PREGNANCY

The American College of Obstetricians and Gynecologists (ACOG) recommends that pregnant women perform up to 30 minutes or more of moderate intensity exercise daily (when possible). It is recommended that the patient consult with her primary provider (M.D., D.O.), or CNM (certified nurse midwife) prior to initiating an exercise program.

ACOG has identified absolute contraindications that will prevent pregnant women from performing aerobic exercise (ACOG 2002). These include:

- Preeclampsia or pregnancy-induced hypertension. Preeclampsia can occur in women with no prenatal history of hypertension or high blood-pressure. Some indicators that a client might have preeclampsia are high blood-pressure or a front headache.

- Second or third trimester bleeding. Bleeding during these trimesters may be indicative of a detaching placenta, placenta previa, or preterm labor. If a client complains of vaginal bleeding she should stop exercise and consult with her primary medical provider.

- Restrictive lung disease. The pregnant woman is now breathing for two. Shortness of breath should be evaluated by a medical provider.

- Hemodynamically significant heart disease. Refer your client to her provider if she experiences an irregular heartbeat, chest pain, or light-headedness.
- Ruptured membranes. There is an increased risk of infection if the pregnant woman's membranes have ruptured.

Other contraindications include an incompetent cervix or cerclage, placenta previa (a low lying placenta) after 26 weeks, and risk for premature labor (ACOG 2002).

The ACOG also recommends that women should stop exercising if they experience any one of the following symptoms: vaginal bleeding, dyspnea prior to exertion, dizziness, headache, chest pain, muscle weakness, calf pain or swelling, preterm labor, decreased fetal movement, or amniotic fluid leakage (ACOG 2002).

Appropriate core exercises for the pregnant client include the following.

- Bridging
- Straight-arm pull-downs
- Side bridge (beginners)

THE CORE AND ATHLETIC PERFORMANCE

The difference between a win and a loss may come down to a matter of inches or seconds. In some cases, the difference between first and second place may be less than a second. What gives the superior athlete or team the advantage? It's usually a mix of great coaching, gifted play, and superior training. Core training plays a crucial role

for athletes who are successful at sports and for those who are able to play injury free.

Core training should be included in a comprehensive training program for all athletes. This section highlights core training for four types of athletes: throwing athletes, swimmers, athletes who swing a racket or bat, and golfers. A sample advanced core training program is provided for each type of athlete. Remember, before beginning an advanced program, most untrained or undertrained athletes should start with basic or intermediate core exercises (see table 9.3).

Throwing

Athletes who perform overhead throwing generate power from the legs and transfer those forces through the torso to the throwing arm. This proximal-to-distal sequencing enables the throwing arm to achieve maximal acceleration at the greatest velocity. Dysfunctional activation of the trunk musculature may result in poorer athletic performance. For example, if a pitcher were to activate his shoulder muscles (the distal segment) before the force contribution of the hip musculature (the proximal segment), the movement pattern would be dysfunctional, and performance would be affected. A dysfunctional trunk also puts the athlete at risk of injuring the throwing arm. A javelin thrower who has a dysfunctional trunk will still attempt to perform at his optimal level on each throw. The athlete will compensate by generating more torque at the shoulder. Repeating this strategy may overload the tissue tolerance at the shoulder or elbow, resulting in a strain or sprain injury to the upper extremity.

Table 9.4 presents a sample core training program for athletes who perform overhead throwing. Strength coaches can make modifications to this training program based on the athlete's sport.

Table 9.3 Sample Core Training Program for the Untrained Athlete

1. Address flexibility limitations.
2. Initiate basic or intermediate core strengthening exercises.
3. Initiate low-intensity sport-specific plyometrics.

Exercise	Sets	Repetitions
Side plank	2-3	10-second holds
Front plank	2-3	10-second holds
Crunches	1-2	10-30
Bridging	1-2	10-30
Overhead ball throws to a rebounder	1-2	20

Table 9.4 Advanced Core Training Program for Athletes Who Perform Overhead Throwing

Exercise	Sets	Repetitions
Lunge	2-3	10-15
Lateral lunge	2-3	10-15
Lunge with ball rotation	2-3	10-15
Standing high-low torso rotations	2-3	20
Shoulder press on a physioball	2-3	10
Side plank with shoulder external rotation	2-3	15

Swimming

To maintain an effective stroke, the swimmer must have a strong core. Strong core muscles will allow the extremities to generate a powerful leg kick and arm stroke. Core weakness, especially in the hips, will affect sport performance and may contribute to the onset of a sport-related injury (Pollard and Fernandez 2004; Allegrucci et al. 1994; Stocker et al. 1995). Swimmers who perform the breaststroke risk injury to the hip adductors due the repetitive adduction motion of the stroke (Grote et al. 2004). To enhance sport performance and reduce the risk of injury, a swimmer should participate in an advanced core training program that incorporates multiplanar movements. Table 9.5 presents an advanced core training program for swimmers.

Racket Sports and Batting

Sports such as tennis and baseball require an athlete to generate significant forces. The athlete must transfer these forces through to the upper extremities to impart force on the ball. However, the swinging motion used in these sports can contribute to the onset of a low back injury. Professional athletes Don Mattingly (baseball) and Andre Agassi (tennis) both suffered from low back pain later in their careers. Core training may help

to reduce the risk of injury to the spine for athletes in these sports.

First, you need to recognize that many athletes may be using poor technique when they are serving in tennis or swinging a bat. In conjunction with any training program you develop for these athletes, each should be seeking help from a professional coach in order to improve technique. When conducting the functional assessment of the athlete, you should give careful consideration to the strength and function of the lower extremities. Dysfunctional activation of the lower extremities may contribute to a low back injury when the athlete uses the back muscles to generate force. Table 9.6 presents an advanced core training program for a tennis or baseball player.

Golf

Injuries to the lumbar spine account for the majority of injuries experienced by golfers. The lumbar spine is at risk because of the various forces—shearing, compressive, torque, and lateral bending forces—created during each golf swing (McHardy et al. 2006; Hosea and Gatt 1996). During each swing, the golfer's lumbar spine experiences compressive loads that are approximately eight times the person's body weight.

Research evidence indicates that golfers who have suffered from LBP demonstrate inadequate

Table 9.5 Advanced Core Training Program for Swimmers

Exercise	Sets	Repetitions
Prone twist	1-2	20-25
Front plank with hip extension (performed bilaterally)	1-2	20-25
Side plank with hip abduction (performed bilaterally)	1-2	20-25
Crunch on the physioball	1-2	20-25
Knee tuck on the physioball	1-2	20-25
Cable torso rotations (low to high and high to low)	1-2	20-25

Table 9.6 Advanced Core Training Program for the Tennis or Baseball Athlete

Exercise	Sets	Repetitions
Lunges	2-3	10-15
Lateral lunge	2-3	10-15
Lunge twist	2-3	10-15
Cable torso rotations (each side)	2-3	10-15
Cable torso rotations (low to high, each side)	2-3	10-15

core strength and endurance (Evans and Oldreive 2000; Evans et al. 2005; Vad et al. 2004). Research reports have identified the transverse abdominis and the trunk rotator muscles as dysfunctional in golfers with low back pain (Evans and Oldreive 2000; Lindsay and Horton 2006). While these particular muscles have been identified as dysfunctional in the literature, you must careful assess endurance capacity and function for all of the core muscles. Table 9.7 contains a sample advanced core training program for golfers. The inclusion of plyometric exercises in the golfer's core program is key to both sport performance and injury prevention (Doan et al. 2006; Fletcher and Hartwell 2004).

When designing training programs for golfers who have suffered from low back pain, you must take the following factors into account: the client's fitness level, the client's training habits (strength and conditioning), the forces exerted on the lumbar spine, and the multiplanar nature of the golf swing (Brumitt and Dale 2008; Coleman and Rankin 2005). Taking these factors into consideration (combined with the findings from the functional assessment) will help you determine the appropriate exercise prescription.

SUMMARY

Including core training in a client's exercise program will help reduce the risk of injury and will improve the client's strength and function (which is especially important for athletes). Core training is also an effective way to continue the functional rehabilitation of the postrehab client.

Arguably, no other region of the body deserves as much attention as the core. The number of individuals who experience back and hip pain indicates the need for the focused prescription of core training exercises. Each year thousands of people require medical attention for injuries that may have been avoided if the person was properly trained. Some of these people will require surgery followed by lengthy rehabilitation and postrehab training. Fitness professionals can positively affect their clients' training and lifestyle habits, helping clients make changes that will reduce the risk of injury and prevent future surgical situations.

Training the core is crucial for all athletes. When athletes fail to train the core, their athletic performance may suffer, and their risk of a sport-related injury may increase.

Table 9.7 Advanced Core Training Program for Golfers (Brumitt and Dale 2008)

Exercise	Sets	Repetitions
Lat pull-downs	3	3-6
Lunge twist	2	15-20
Hang twist	2	15-20
Prone twist	2	15-20
Roman twist	2	15-20
Kettleball squats	2	15-20
Overhead ball throw (plyometric)	1-3	10
Standing horizontal throws (each side)	1-3	10
Seated horizontal throws (each side)	1-3	10

Glossary

abdominal brace—An isometric cocontraction of the abdominal wall and the posterior torso muscles that is performed to enhance spine stability.

active range of motion (AROM)—Refers to the range of motion through which an individual can actively move a joint using his or her muscles.

adduction—The process of moving an extremity (or joint) toward the middle of the body.

body mass index (BMI)—A measurement tool developed to compare a person's weight to the person's height. Results of this measurement are used as a preliminary diagnostic tool for obesity.

concomitant—Occurring at the same time; in medicine, this term relates to two or more conditions experienced by the patient at one time.

core training—Training programs consisting of exercises that address the muscles of the spine, the abdominal region, and the hips.

disc protrusion—An injury in which the inner portion of the disc bulges toward the periphery, pushing against the outer portion of the disc without disruption of the disc.

disc sequestration—An injury in which the inner portion of the disc is disrupted and becomes separated from the disc.

discectomy—Surgical procedure performed to excise (remove) a portion of a herniated intervertebral disc.

dynamic flexibility—Refers to the range of motion demonstrated by a client when performing any active motion.

epidemiological—Relating to epidemiology, which is the study of the distribution and causes of disease and illness within the population.

ergonomics—The field of study related to the evaluation of work settings and the subsequent changes made to work sites to improve workers' safety and performance.

evidence based—Relating to the practice of evidence-based medicine. The practice of evidence-based medicine refers to a health care provider using the best available research, his or her own clinical experience, and the patient's values when determining the best treatment approach for the patient.

Fairbank's sign—A manually performed musculoskeletal medical test reported to assess the mobility of the patella.

flexibility—Refers to the ability to demonstrate movement about a joint or a series of joints and the associated soft tissues; a person's ability to move through the available range of motion.

functional test—A physical test performed to identify dysfunctional movement patterns.

ginglymoid—An object or structure that looks like a hinge; the knee and the elbow are ginglymoid (hinge joints).

goniometer—A device used to measure the degree of motion available at a joint.

handheld dynamometer—A handheld device that provides a reliable quantitative measure of a person's muscular strength.

hypermobile—Range of motion at a joint that is greater or more excessive than the population norms.

hypomobile—Range of motion at a joint that is less than the population norms.

idiopathic—Having no known cause.

iliotibial band syndrome (ITBS)—A syndrome associated with pain at the lateral (outer) knee or lateral thigh. The iliotibial band is a thick tissue extending from the lateral hip to the lateral knee. This syndrome is often brought on by overuse or by changes in training associated with running or cycling.

inferior—When referring to a location on the body, the inferior body part is located below (or closer to the ground) than another body part or region.

intermittent—Occurring at different periods of time; in regard to pain, intermittent means that the pain is not consistent in nature.

internal rotation—Rotation of an extremity about its axis of rotation toward the middle or midline of the body.

kinetic link principle—The biomechanical relationship describing the interrelated nature of successive joint segments in the human body.

kyphosis—An abnormal or excessive posterior curvature of the spine; primarily occurs in the thoracic spine.

laxity—Excessive play, or movement, created at a joint.

lordosis—An abnormal or excessive anterior curvature of the spine; primarily occurs in the lumbar spine.

mechanical model—One of two theoretical models describing how plyometric training improves functional power. The other model is the neurophysiological model.

medial tibial stress syndrome (MTSS)—A pain syndrome occurring in the leg and brought on by exercise. One or more biomechanical causes can contribute to this condition.

modalities—A general term used to describe equipment (e.g., electrical stimulation or ultrasound) used in a rehabilitation setting in order to provide a therapeutic effect to the patient.

muscle spindle—A proprioceptive organ aligned between muscle fibers. The muscle spindle responds to the speed and degree of a stretch to the muscle.

neurophysiological model—One of two theoretical models describing how plyometric training improves functional power. The other model is the mechanical model.

pars interarticularis—Posterior component of a vertebra, may be subject to injury.

passive range of motion (PROM)—Refers to the degree of passive motion (motion that is not influenced by the person's volitional control) available at a joint.

paucity—A lack of or a scarcity. A paucity of research denotes a lack of available research (or a minimal amount of research) related to the topic in question.

posterior—Located behind something or located to the back of the body.

postrehab—Refers to patients who have completed formal clinical rehabilitation but have not completely returned to their preinjured or optimal status.

potentiation—The resulting enhanced effect when one object or event is combined with another.

proprioception—The ability to sense or perceive movement of the body and its orientation in space.

proximal-to-distal sequencing—Refers to how a force may be generated and then transferred through the body. For example, as a baseball pitcher begins his windup, he is generating a force with his rear leg. During the pitching motion, this force is transferred from the lower extremity (proximally) through the body to the throwing arm (distally) in order to maximize the velocity of the pitch.

quadruped—A position in which a client supports her body with both hands and knees resting on the surface.

range of motion (ROM)—The degree of motion available at a joint.

rebounder—A piece of training equipment consisting of a flexible, trampoline-like netting that may be manipulated to assume a variety of angular positions in space. This machine is often used to improve power or to aid rehabilitation.

reliable—A test (medical or functional) is considered reliable if it yields similar results consistently.

series elastic component (SEC)—An anatomic structure consisting of a tendon and the associated connective tissue.

static flexibility—The range of motion that can be demonstrated at a joint without any muscular activation.

supraphysiologic—Refers to an amount (force or load) that is above what the tissue can safely experience.

trigger points—Tight and painful points within a muscle, common among people who suffer from back or shoulder pain.

valgus—An abnormal alignment of a limb; the limb is bent away (outward) from the midline of the body.

valid—A test (medical or functional) is considered valid if it measures what it is intended to measure.

References

Chapter 1

Brown, K. 2004. One-on-one. Compliance: The phenomenon of giving up. *Strength and Conditioning Journal* 26(3): 68-69.

Chiu, L.Z.F. 2007. Are specific spine stabilization exercises necessary for athletes? *Strength and Conditioning Journal* 29(1): 15-17.

Fredericson M, Cookingham C.L., Chaudhari A.M., Dowdell B.C., Oestreicher N, and S.A. Sahrmann. 2000. Hip abductor weakness in distance runners with iliotibial band syndrome. *Clinical Journal of Sports Medicine* 10(3): 169-175.

Jaramillo, J., T.W. Worrell, and C.D. Ingersoll. 1994. Hip isometric strength following knee surgery. *Journal of Orthopaedic and Sports Physical Therapy* 20(3): 160-165.

Katz, J.N. 2006. Lumbar disc disorders and low-back pain: socioeconomic factors and consequences. *Journal of Bone and Joint Surgery (Am)* 88 Suppl 2: 21-24.

Kibler, W.B. 1998. The role of the scapula in athletic shoulder function. *American Journal of Sports Medicine* 26(2): 325-337.

Kibler, W.B., J. Press, and A. Sciascia. 2006. The role of core stability in athletic function. *Sports Medicine* 36(3): 189-198.

Leetun D.T., M.L. Ireland, J.D. Willson, B.T. Ballantyne, and M. Davis. 2004. Core stability measures as risk factors for lower extremity injury in athletes. *Medicine and Science in Sports and Exercise* 36(6): 926-934.

Luo, X., R. Pietrobon, S.X. Sun, G.G. Liu, and L. Hey. 2004. Estimates and patterns of direct health care expenditures among individuals with back pain in the United States. *Spine* 29(1): 79-86.

McGill, S. 2002. *Low back disorders: Evidence-based prevention and rehabilitation.* Champaign, IL: Human Kinetics.

Middleton, A. 2004. Chronic low back pain: Patient compliance with physiotherapy advice and exercise, perceived barriers and motivation. *Physical Therapy Reviews* 9(3): 153-160.

Milne, M., C. Hall, and L. Forwell. 2005. Self-efficacy, imagery use, and adherence to rehabilitation by injured athletes. *Journal of Sport Rehabilitation* 14(2): 150-167.

Muse, T. 2005. Motivation and adherence to exercise for older adults. *Topics in Geriatric Rehabilitation* 21(2): 107-115.

Nadler, S.F., G.A. Malanga., M. DePrince, T.P. Stitik, and J.H. Feinberg. 2000. The relationship between lower extremity injury, low back pain, and hip muscle strength in male and female collegiate athletes. *Clinical Journal of Sports Medicine* 10(2): 89-97.

Nadler, S.F., G.A. Malanga, J.H. Feinberg, M. Prybicien, T.P. Stitik, and M. Deprince. 2001. Relationship between hip muscle imbalance and occurrence of low back pain in collegiate athletes: a prospective study. *American Journal of Physical Medicine and Rehabilitation* 80(8): 572-577.

Niemuth, P.E., R.J. Johnson, M.J. Myers, and T.J. Thieman. 2005. Hip muscle weakness and overuse injuries in recreational runners. *Clinical Journal of Sport Medicine* 15(1): 14-21.

Plisky, M.S., M.J. Rauh, B. Heiderscheit, F.B. Underwood, and R.T. Tank. 2007. Medial tibial stress syndrome in high school cross-country runners: incidence and risk factors. *Journal of Orthopaedic and Sports Physical Therapy* 37(2): 40-47.

Rauh, M.J., T.D. Koepsell, F.P. Rivara, A.J. Margherita, and S.G. Rice. 2006. Epidemiology of musculoskeletal injuries among high school cross-country runners. *American Journal of Epidemiology* 163(2): 151-159.

Rauh, M.J., A.J. Margherita, S.G. Rice, T.D. Koepsell, and F.P. Rivara. 2000. High school cross country running injuries: A longitudinal study. *Clinical Journal of Sport Medicine* 10(2): 110-116.

Rasmussen-Barr, E., Nilsson-Wikmar, L., & Arvidsson, I. 2003. Stabilizing training compared with manual treatment in sub-acute and chronic low-back pain. *Manual Therapy* 8(4), 233-241.

Sabin, K.L. 2005. Older adults and motivations for therapy and exercise: Issues, influences, and interventions. *Topics in Geriatric Rehabilitation* 21(3): 215-220.

Vad, V.B., A.L. Bhat, D. Basrai, A. Gebeh, D.D. Aspergren, and J.R. Andrews. 2004. Low back pain in professional golfers: the role of associated hip and low back range-of-motion deficits. *American Journal of Sports Medicine* 32(2): 494-497.

Chapter 2

Behnke, R. 2006. *Kinetic anatomy.* 2nd ed. Champaign, IL: Human Kinetics.

Bogduk, N. 2005. *Clinical anatomy of the lumbar spine and sacrum.* 4th ed. New York: Elsevier.

Ellenbecker, T.S., and G.J. Davies. 2001. *Closed kinetic chain exercises: A comprehensive guide to multiple joint exercises.* Champaign, IL: Human Kinetics.

Katz, J.N. 2006. Lumbar disc disorders and low-back pain: socioeconomic factors and consequences. *Journal of Bone and Joint Surgery (Am)* 88(Suppl 2): 21-24.

Khaund, R., and S.H. Flynn. 2005. Iliotibial band syndrome: A common source of knee pain. *American Family Physician* 71: 1545-1550.

Kibler, W.B. 1994. Clinical biomechanics of the elbow in tennis: Implications for evaluation and diagnosis. *Medicine and Science in Sports and Exercise* 26(10): 1203-1206.

Kibler, W.B., J. Press, and A. Sciascia. 2006. The role of core stability in athletic function. *Sports Medicine* 36(3): 189-198.

Luo, X., Pietrobon, R., Sun, S.X., Liu, G.G., and L. Hey. 2004. Estimates and patterns of direct health care expenditures among individuals with back pain in the United States. *Spine* 29(1): 79-86.

McGill, S. 2002. *Low back disorders: Evidence-based prevention and rehabilitation.* Champaign, IL: Human Kinetics.

Neumann, D.A. 2002. *Kinesiology of the musculoskeletal system: Foundations for physical rehabilitation.* St. Louis: Mosby.

Niemuth, P.E., R.J. Johnson, M.J. Myers, and T.J. Thieman. 2005. Hip muscle weakness and overuse injuries in recreational runners. *Clinical Journal of Sport Medicine* 15(1): 14-21.

Powers, C.M. 2003. The influence of altered lower-extremity kinematics on patellofemoral joint dysfunction: A theoretical perspective. *Journal of Orthopaedic and Sports Physical Therapy* 33(11): 639-646.

Rasmussen-Barr, E., L. Nilsson-Wikmar, and I. Arvidsson. 2003. Stabilizing training compared with manual treatment in sub-acute and chronic low-back pain. *Manual Therapy* 8(4), 233-241.

Richardson, C., G. Jull, P. Hodges, and J. Hides. 1999. *Therapeutic exercise for spinal segmental stabilization in low back pain: Scientific basis and clinical approach.* New York: Churchill Livingstone.

Roetert, E.P., T.S. Ellenbecker, D.A. Chu, and B.S. Bugg. 1997. Tennis-specific shoulder and trunk strength training. *Strength and Conditioning Journal* 19(3): 31-43.

Trainor, T.J., and S.W. Wiesel. 2002. Epidemiology of back pain in the athlete. *Clinical Sports Medicine* 21(1): 93-103.

Travell, J.G., and D.G. Simons. 1983. *Myofascial pain and dysfunction: The trigger point manual.* Vol. 1. Baltimore: Williams & Wilkins.

Young, J.L., J.M. Press, and S.A. Herring. 1997. The disc at risk in athletes: Perspectives on operative and nonoperative care. *Medicine and Science in Sports and Exercise* 29(7): 222-232.

Chapter 3

Jamnik, V.K., N. Gledhill, and R.J. Shephard. 2007. Revised clearance for participation in physical activity: greater screening responsibility for qualified university-educated fitness professionals. *Applied Physiology, Nutrition, and Metabolism* 32(6): 1191-1197.

McGill, S. 2002. *Low back disorders: Evidence-based prevention and rehabilitation.* Champaign, IL: Human Kinetics.

Shephard, R.J. 1988. PAR-Q, Canadian home fitness test and exercise screening alternatives. *Sports Medicine* 5(3): 185-195.

Thomas, S., J. Reading, and R.J. Shephard. 1992. Revision of the physical activity readiness questionnaire (PAR_Q). *Canadian Journal of Sports Sciences* 17(4): 338-345.

Chapter 4

Biering-Sorensen, F. 1984. Physical measurements as risk indicators for low-back trouble over a one-year period. *Spine* 9: 106-119.

DiMattia, M.A., A.L. Livengood, T.L. Uhl, C.G. Mattacola, and T.R. Malone. 2005. What are the validity of the single-leg-squat test and its relationship to hip-abduction strength? *Journal of Sport Rehabilitation* 14: 108-123.

Gao, X., D. Gordon, D. Zhang, R. Browne, C. Helms, J. Gillum, S. Weber, S. Devroy, S. Swaney, M. Dobbs, J. Morcuende, V. Sheffield, M. Lovett, A. Bowcock, J. Herring, and C. Wise. 2007. CHD7 gene polymorphisms are associated with susceptibility to idiopathic scoliosis. *American Journal of Human Genetics* 80(5): 957-965.

Gribble, P. 2003. The star excursion balance tests as a measurement tool. *Athletic Therapy Today* 8(2): 46-47.

Jewell, D.V. 2008. *Guide to evidence-based physical therapy practice.* Sudbury, MA: Jones and Bartlett.

Livengood, A.L., M.A. DiMattia, and T.L. Uhl. 2004. "Dynamic trendelenburg": Single-leg-squat test for gluteus medius strength. *Athletic Therapy Today* 9(1): 24-25.

McGill, S. 2002. *Low back disorders: Evidence-based prevention and rehabilitation.* Champaign, IL: Human Kinetics.

Plastaras, C.T., J.D. Rittenberg, K.E. Rittenberg, J. Press, and V. Akuthota. 2005. Comprehensive functional evaluation of the injured runner. *Physical Medicine and Rehabilitation Clinics of North America* 16: 623-649.

Plisky, P.J., M.J. Rauh, T.W. Kaminski, and F.B. Underwood. 2006. Star excursion balance test as a predictor of lower extremity injury in high school basketball players. *Journal of Orthopaedic Sports Physical Therapy* 36(12): 911-919.

Portney, L.G., and M.P. Watkins. 1999. *Foundations of clinical research: Applications to practice.* 2nd ed. Norwalk, CT: Appleton & Lange.

Zeller, B.L., J.L. McCrory, W.B. Kibler, and T.L. Uhl. 2003. Differences in kinematics and electromyographic activity between men and women during the single-legged squat. *American Journal of Sports Medicine* 31: 449-456.

Chapter 5

Alaranta, H., S. Luoto, M. Heliovaara, and H. Hurri. 1995. Static back endurance and the risk of low-back pain. *Clinical Biomechanics* 10(6): 323-324.

Baechle, T.R., R.W. Earle, and D. Wathen. 2000. Resistance training. In T.R. Baechle and R.W. Earle (Eds.), *Essentials of strength training and conditioning.* 2nd ed. Champaign, IL: Human Kinetics.

Biering-Sorensen, F. 1984. Physical measurements as risk indicators for low-back trouble over a one-year period. *Spine* 9: 106-119.

Doan, B.K., R.U. Newton, Y.H. Kwon, and W.J. Kraemer. 2006. Effects of physical conditioning on intercollegiate golfer performance. *Journal of Strength and Conditioning Research* 20(1): 62-72.

Fletcher, I.M., and M. Hartwell. 2004. Effect of an 8-week combined weights and plyometrics training program on golf drive performance. *Journal of Strength and Conditioning Research* 18(1): 59-62.

McGill, S. 2002. *Low back disorders: Evidence-based prevention and rehabilitation.* Champaign, IL: Human Kinetics.

McGill, S. 2004. *Ultimate back fitness and performance.* Ontario, Canada: Wabano.

Myer, G.D., Ford, K.R., Brent, J.L., and T.E. Hewett. 2006. The effects of plyometric vs. dynamic stabilization and balance training on power, balance, and landing force in female athletes. *Journal of Strength and Conditioning Research* 20(2): 345-353.

Myer, G.D., Chu, D.A., Brent, J.L., and T.E. Hewett. 2008. Trunk and hip control neuromuscular training for the prevention of knee joint injury. *Clinics in Sports Medicine.* 27(3): 425-448.

Wathen, D., T.R. Baechle, and R.W. Earle. 2000. Training variation: Periodization. In T.R. Baechle and R.W. Earle (Eds.), *Essentials of strength training and conditioning.* 2nd ed. Champaign, IL: Human Kinetics.

Chapter 6

Chu, D.A., and D.J. Cordier. 2000. Plyometrics in rehabilitation. In T.S. Ellenbecker, *Knee ligament rehabilitation.* New York: Churchill Livingstone.

McGill, S.M. 2002. *Low back disorders: Evidence-based prevention and rehabilitation.* Champaign, IL: Human Kinetics.

McGill, S.M. 2004. *Ultimate back fitness and performance.* Waterloo, Ontario, Canada: Wabuno.

Chapter 7

Alter, M.J. 2004. *Science of flexibility.* 3rd ed. Champaign, IL: Human Kinetics.

Bandy, W.D., J.M. Irion, and M. Briggler. 1994. The effect of time on static stretch on the flexibility of the hamstring muscles. *Physical Therapy* 74(9): 845-852.

Bannerman, N., E. Pentecost, S. Rutter, S. Willoughby, and A. Vujnovich. 1996. Increase in soleus muscle length: A comparison between two stretching techniques. *New Zealand Journal of Physiotherapy* 24(3): 15-18.

Barlow, A., R. Clarke, N. Johnson, B. Seabourne, D. Thomas, and J. Gal. 2004. Effect of massage on the hamstring muscle group on performance of the sit and reach test. *British Journal of Sports Medicine* 38: 349-351.

Beedle, B.B., and C.L. Mann. 2007. A comparison of two warm-ups on joint range of motion. *Journal of Strength and Conditioning Research* 21(3): 776-779.

Boyle, K.L., P. Witt, and C. Riegger-Krugh. 2003. Intra-rater and inter-rater reliability of the Beighton and Horan joint mobility index. *Journal of Athletic Training* 38: 281-285.

Bradley, P.S., P.D. Olsen, and M.D. Portas. 2007. The effect of static, ballistic, and proprioceptive neuromuscular facilitation stretching on vertical jump performance. *Journal of Strength and Conditioning Research* 21(1): 223-226.

Brumitt, J. 2008. The role of massage in sports performance and rehabilitation: Current evidence and future direction. *North American Journal of Sports Physical Therapy* 3(1): 7-21.

Clark, M.A., and A. Russell. 2002. *Optimum performance training for the performance enhancement specialist: Home study course.* Thousand Oaks, CA: National Academy of Sports Medicine.

Decoster, L.C., J. Cleland, C. Altieri, and P. Russell. 2005. The effect of hamstring stretching on range of motion: A systematic literature review. *Journal of Orthopaedic and Sports Physical Therapy* 35: 377-387.

Faigenbaum, A.D., M. Belluci, A. Bernieri, B. Bakker, and K. Hoorens. 2005. Acute effects of different warm-up protocols on fitness performance in children. *Journal of Strength and Conditioning Research* 19(2): 376-381.

Fredericson, M., J.J. White, J.M. MacMahon, and T.P. Andriacchi. 2002. Quantitative analysis of the relative effectiveness of 3 iliotibial band stretches. *Archives of Physical Medicine and Rehabilitation* 83: 589-592.

Hendrick, A. 2000. Dynamic flexibility training. *Strength and Conditioning Journal* 22(5): 33-38.

Hewett, T.E., T.N. Lindenfeld, J.V. Riccobene, and F.R. Noyes. 1999. The effect of neuromuscular training on the incidence of knee injury in female athletes: A prospective study. *American Journal of Sports Medicine* 27(6): 699-706.

Holcomb, W.R. 2000. Stretching and warm-up. In T.R. Baechle and R.W. Earle (Eds.), *Essentials of strength training and conditioning.* 2nd ed. Champaign, IL: Human Kinetics.

Hopper, D., M. Conneely, F. Chromiak, E. Canini, J. Berggren, and K. Briffa. 2005. Evaluation of the effect of two massage techniques on hamstring muscle length in competitive female hockey players. *Physical Therapy in Sport* 6: 137-145.

Jeffreys, I. 2008. Warm-up and stretching. Chap. 13 in T.R. Baechle and R.W. Earle (Eds.), *Essentials of strength training and conditioning.* 3rd ed. Champaign, IL: Human Kinetics.

Kaltenborn, J.M. 2006. The foam roll: A complement to any therapy. *Athletic Therapy Today* 11(1): 38-39.

LaRoche, D.P., and D.A.J. Connolly. 2006. Effects of stretching on passive muscle tension and response to eccentric exercise. *American Journal of Sports Medicine* 34(6): 1000-1007.

Little, T., and A.G. Williams. 2006. Effects of differential stretching protocols during warm-ups on high-speed motor capacities in professional soccer players. *Journal of Strength and Conditioning Research* 20(1): 203-207.

Mangine, G.T., N.A. Ratamess, J.R. Hoffman, A.D. Faigenbaum, J. Kang, and A. Chilakos. 2008. The effects of combined ballistic and heavy resistance training on maximal lower- and upper-body strength in recreationally trained men. *Journal of Strength and Conditioning Research* 22(1): 132-139.

Messier, S.P., D.G. Edwards, and D.F. Martin. 1995. Clinical investigations: Etiology of iliotibial band friction syndrome in distance runners. *Medicine and Science in Sports and Exercise* 27(7): 951-960.

Nelson, A.G., J. Kokkonen, and D.A. Arnall. 2005. Acute muscle stretching inhibits muscle strength endurance performance. *Journal of Strength and Conditioning Research* 19(2): 338-343.

Paluska, S.A. 2005. An overview of hip injuries in running. *Sports Medicine* 35(11): 991-1014.

Rubini, E.C., A.L.L. Costa, and P.S.C. Gomes. 2007. The effects of stretching on strength performance. *Sports Medicine* 37(3): 213-224.

Stone, M., M.W. Ramsey, A.M. Kinser, H.S. O'Bryant, C. Ayers, and W.A. Sands. 2006. Stretching: Acute and chronic? The potential consequences. *Strength and Conditioning Journal* 28(6): 66-74.

Unick, J., H.S. Kieffer, W. Cheesman, and A. Feeney. 2005. The acute effects of static and ballistic stretching on vertical jump performance in trained women. *Journal of Strength and Conditioning Research* 19(1) (February): 206-212.

Woods, K., P. Bishop, and E. Jones. 2007. Warm-up and stretching in the prevention of muscular injury. *Sports Medicine* 37(12): 1089-1099.

Woolstenhulme, M.T., C.M. Griffiths, E.M. Woolstenhulme, and A.C. Parcell. 2006. Ballistic stretching increases flexibility and acute jump height when combined with basketball activity. *Journal of Strength and Conditioning Research* 20(4): 799-803.

Yamaguchi, T., and K. Ishii. 2005. Effects of static stretching for 30 seconds and dynamic stretching on leg extension power. *Journal of Strength and Conditioning Research* 19(3): 677-683.

Yamaguchi, T., K. Ishii, M. Yamanaka, and K. Yasuda. 2006. Acute effect of static stretching on power output during concentric dynamic constant external resistance leg extension. *Journal of Strength and Conditioning Research* 20(4): 804-810.

Chapter 8

Allerheiligen, B., and R. Rogers. 1995. Plyometrics program design, part 2. *NSCA Journal* 17(5): 33-39.

Chu, D.A. 1998. *Jumping into plyometrics*. 2nd ed. Champaign, IL: Human Kinetics.

Chu, D.A. 2001. Point/counterpoint: Plyometrics or not?—Counterpoint. *Strength and Conditioning Journal* 23(2): 71-72.

Chu, D.A., and D.J. Cordier. 2000. Plyometrics in rehabilitation. In T.S. Ellenbecker, *Knee ligament rehabilitation*. New York: Churchill Livingstone.

Doan, B.K., R.U. Newton, Y.H. Kwon, and W.J. Kraemer. 2006. Effects of physical conditioning on intercollegiate golfer performance. *Journal of Strength and Conditioning Research* 20(1): 62-72.

Fletcher, I.M., and M. Hartwell. 2004. Effect of an 8-week combined weights and plyometrics training program on golf drive performance. *Journal of Strength and Conditioning Research* 18(1): 59-62.

Harman, E. 2000. The biomechanics of resistance exercise. In T.R. Baechle and R.W. Earle (Eds.), *Essentials of strength training and conditioning*. 2nd ed. Champaign, IL: Human Kinetics.

Hewett, T.E., T.N. Lindenfeld, J.V. Riccobene, and F.R. Noyes. 1999. The effect of neuromuscular training on the incidence of knee injury in female athletes: A prospective study. *American Journal of Sports Medicine* 27(6): 699-706.

Hewett, T.E., A.L. Stroupe, T.A. Nance, and F.R. Noyes. 1996. Plyometric training in female athletes: Decreased impact forces and increased hamstring torques. *American Journal of Sports Medicine* 24(6): 765-773.

Holcomb, W.R., D.M. Kleiner, and D.A. Chu. 1998. Plyometrics: considerations for safe and effective training. *Strength and Conditioning Journal* 20(3): 36-39.

Knuttgen, H., and W. Kraemer. 1987. Terminology and measurement in exercise performance. *Journal of Applied Sport Science Research* 1(1): 1-10.

National Strength and Conditioning Association. 1993. *National Strength and Conditioning Journal* 15(3):16.

Potach, D.H., and D.A. Chu. 2000. Plyometric training. In T.R. Baechle and R.W. Earle (Eds.), *Essentials of strength training and conditioning*. 2nd ed. Champaign, IL: Human Kinetics.

Radcliffe, J.C., and R.C. Farentinos. 1999. *High-powered plyometrics*. Champaign, IL: Human Kinetics.

Stone, M.H., and H.S. O'Bryant. 1987. *Weight training: A scientific approach*. Minneapolis: Bellwether Press.

Wathen, D. 1993. Literature review: plyometric exercise. *National Strength and Conditioning Journal* 15(3): 17-19.

Chapter 9

Allegrucci, M., S.L. Whitney, and J.J. Irrgang. 1994. Clinical implications of secondary impingement of the shoulder in freestyle swimmers. *Journal of Orthopaedic Sports Physical Therapy* 20(6): 307-318.

ACOG Committee on Obstetric Practice. 2002. ACOG Committee Opinion. Number 267, January 2002: Exercise during pregnancy and the postpartum period. *Obstetrics and Gynecology* 99: 171-173.

Anderson, K., S.M. Strickland, and R. Warren. 2001. Hip and groin injuries in athletes. *American Journal of Sports Medicine* 29(4): 521-533.

Brumitt, J., and R.B. Dale. 2008. Functional rehabilitation exercise prescription for golfers. *Athletic Therapy Today* 13(2): 37-41.

Coleman, S.C., and A.J. Rankin. 2005. A three-dimensional examination of the planar nature of the golf swing. *Journal of Sports Sciences* 23(3): 227-234.

Doan, B., R. Newton, Y. Kwon, and W. Kraemer. 2006. Effects of physical conditioning on intercollegiate golfer performance. *Journal of Strength and Conditioning Research* 20(1): 62-72.

Evans, C., and W. Oldreive. 2000. A study to investigate whether golfers with a history of low back pain show a reduced endurance of transversus abdominis. *Journal of Manipulative and Physiological Therapeutics* 8(4): 162-174.

Evans, K., K. Refshauge, R. Adams, and L. Aliprandi. 2005. Predictors of low back pain in young elite golfers: A preliminary study. *Physical Therapy in Sport* 6(3): 122-130.

Fletcher, I., and M. Hartwell. 2004. Effect of an 8-week combined weights and plyometric training program on golf drive performance. *Journal of Strength and Conditioning Research* 18(1): 59-62.

Grote, K., T.L. Lincoln, and J.G. Gamble. 2004. Hip adductor injury in competitive swimmers. *American Journal of Sports Medicine* 32(1): 104-108.

Hosea, T.M., and C.J. Gatt Jr. 1996. Back pain in golf. *Clinics in Sports Medicine* 15(1): 37-53.

Lindsay, D., and J. Horton. 2006. Comparison of spine motion in elite golfers with and without low back pain. *North American Journal of Sports Physical Therapy* 1(2): 80-89.

McHardy, A., H. Pollard, and K. Luo. 2006. Golf injuries: A review of the literature. *Sports Medicine* 36(2): 171-187.

Ostelo, R.W., H.C. de Vet, G. Waddell, M.R. Kerckhoffs, P. Leffers, and M. van Tulder. 2003. Rehabilitation following first-time disc surgery: A systematic review within the framework of the Cochrane collaboration. *Spine* 28(3): 209-218.

Pollard, H., and M. Fernandez. 2004. Spinal musculoskeletal injuries associated with swimming: A discussion of technique. *Australasian Chiropractic and Osteopathy* 12(2): 72-80.

Rasmussen-Barr, E., L. Nilsson-Wikmar, and I. Arvidsson. 2003. Stabilizing training compared with manual treatment in sub-acute and chronic low-back pain. *Manual Therapy* 8(4): 233-241.

Stocker, D., M. Pink, and F.W. Jobe. 1995. Comparison of shoulder injury in collegiate- and master's-level swimmers. *Clinical Journal of Sport Medicine* 5(1): 4-8.

Tyler, T.F., S.J. Nicholas, R.J. Campbell, S. Donellan, and M.P. McHugh. 2002. The effectiveness of a preseason exercise program to prevent adductor muscle strains in professional hockey players. *American Journal of Sports Medicine* 30(5): 680-683.

Tyler, T.F., S.J. Nicholas, R.J. Campbell, and M.P. McHugh. 2001. The association of hip strength and flexibility with the incidence of adductor muscle strains in professional ice hockey players. *American Journal of Sports Medicine* 29(2): 124-128.

Vad, V.B., A.L. Bhat, D. Basrai, A. Gebeh, D.D. Aspergren, and J.R. Andrews. 2004. Low back pain in professional golfers: The role of associated hip and low back range-of-motion deficits. *American Journal of Sports Medicine* 32(2): 494-497.

Index

Note: The italicized *f* and *t* following page numbers refer to figures and tables, respectively.

About the Contributor

Jason Brumitt, MSPT, SCS, ATC, CSCS*D, is an instructor of physical therapy at Pacific University in Hillsboro, Oregon. He earned his master of science degree in physical therapy from Pacific University and is currently a doctoral candidate at Rocky Mountain University of Health Professions. Brumitt is board certified in sports physical therapy and certified as an athletic trainer. He is also a certified strength and conditioning specialist with distinction. In addition to his teaching responsibilities, he provides clinical rehabilitation services to the student-athletes of Pacific University.

Brumitt is the author of "Ounce of Prevention," a regularly featured column in the National Strength and Conditioning Association's (NSCA) *Performance Training Journal.* He has published numerous articles on sports medicine and strength training in the *North American Journal of Sports Physical Therapy,* the *New Zealand Journal of Physiotherapy, Physiotherapy Theory and Practice, Strength and Conditioning Journal,* and *Athletic Therapy Today.* Brumitt has presented lectures on core training at local and national professional conferences as an invited speaker for both the NSCA and the Northwest Athletic Trainers' Association (NWATA).

Brumitt, his wife, and their three children reside in Damascus, Oregon.

DVD Menu

Physical Assessment and Functional Testing

Plumb Line Test

Active Range of Motion Testing of the Spine—Rotation

Hip Crossover Test

Squat Assessment

Lunge Assessment

Single-Leg Squat Test

Star Excursion Balance Test

Hip Passive Range of Motion—Internal Rotation

Hip Passive Range of Motion—External Rotation

Straight Leg Raise Test

Thomas Test

Ober's Test

Core Exercises

Abdominal Bracing

Finding Neutral Spine in Quadruped

Straight Leg Raise

Bridging With a March

Bridging With Leg Extension

Lunge Twist

Backward Lunge

Lunge with Ball Rotation

Chu's Lunge Series for Athletes

Standing High-Low Torso Rotations

Over-Unders

Hip Crossover

Knee Tuck on a Physioball

Ball Plank Twists

Bench Press on a Physioball

Shoulder Press on a Physioball

Jackknife on a Physioball

Inverted Hamstring

Hang Twist

Prone Twist

V-Ups

Side Bridge With Shoulder External Rotation

Three-Point Plank With Upper Extremity Exercise

Roman Twist

Russian Twist

Russian Twist on a Physioball

Romanian Deadlift

Pull-Up

Seated Row

Cable Diagonal Patterns

Core Flexibility

Crossover Toe Touch

Contract Relax Stretch for the Hamstrings

Hold-Relax With Agonist Contraction Stretch for the Hamstrings

Foam Roll Application for the Hamstrings

Foam Roll Application for the Quadriceps

Trail Leg Walking

Foam Roll Application for the Iliotibial Band

Foam Roll Application for the Gluteus Maximus

Foam Roll Application for the Hip Adductors

Kneeling Side Lunge

Side Lunge Stretch

Foam Roll Application for the Piriformis

Foam Roll Application for the Muscles of the Low Back

Foam Roll Application for the Latissimus Dorsi

Plyometric Training

Underhand Throw

Overhead Throw

Trunk Rotation

Side Throw

Backward Throw

Medicine Ball Seated Side Throw

Medicine Ball Reach-Ups

Pull-Over Pass

Medicine Ball Sit-Up

Twist and Touch

Sit-Up and Throw

Vertical Swing

Medicine Ball Scoop Toss

Credits